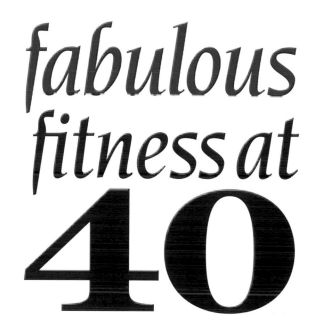

# *fabulous fitness at* 40

The fitness guru's guide to transforming
your life through mastering
your mind and body

## Ladan Soltani

**Fabulous Fitness at 40**
The fitness guru's guide to transforming your life through mastering your mind and body
© Ladan Soltani

ISBN: 978-1-906316-61-7

Published in 2011 by HotHive Books, Evesham, UK.
www.thehothive.com

The right of Ladan Soltani to be identified as the author of this work has been asserted
by her in accordance with the Copyright, Designs and Patents Act 1988.

A CIP record of this book is available from the British Library.

Printed in the UK by Cambrian Printers.

# Health Warning

Before participating in this exercise programme, please consult your doctor.

Do not use this exercise programme if you are pregnant, injured or have a medical condition, or are over the age of 65.

If you are feeling at all unwell, have recently eaten a heavy meal, have been drinking alcohol or if you are taking any drugs without first having consulted your doctor, abstain from using this exercise programme.

If you experience dizziness, shortness of breath, fainting or bleeding do not attempt to do any of these exercises. Consult a medical practitioner immediately.

The reader accepts all responsibility for their health and any resultant injury or mishap that may affect their wellbeing or health in any way. The reader holds harmless of any responsibility the instructor, facility or any persons involved with this programme.

The creators, producers and distributors of this book do not accept responsibility for any injury or accident incurred as a result of following the exercises in the programmes.

To all my enthusiastic and devoted class participants:

I am sincerely grateful for your kind words in which you mention that I made a difference to your life, health and wellbeing; just as you have to mine in another way.

This book is dedicated to you...

# Acknowledgements

First of all, I would like to thank my publisher, Karen Swinden, for having faith and belief in me. It feels amazing to be given this opportunity to get my message out there so I can help those who are searching for a deeper connection within themselves. You don't know how happy this makes me.

A huge thanks also goes to Greg and Anna from 'bodyinbalance' Sky TV channel for their help and advice in making a TV series of this book.

I would like to thank Rebecca Curran for the wonderful pictures in this book and its associated DVD. It has been great fun working with you.

My sincere gratitude to all my sponsors: Serena for kindly donating clothing from 'rockwear' and her own brand 'stepnpump' (www.stepnpump.com), and John for the fitness equipment from physical company (www.physicalcompany. co.uk).

Thank you to my great teachers of Sivananda yoga, and Clayton Horton from Green Path Yoga in San Francisco for carrying through the wonderful works of the yoga lineage.

Thanks also go to all my dear friends and family who have supported me through this and believed in me. In particular, Aunty Suzy, Ana, Michael, Debs, Tim, Chris, Helen, Kat, Oz and Sabrina for being there for me and most importantly for your fantastic friendships. I'm glad I met all of you.

I personally thank Corinne Blum and Lisa Smith for coming into my life. Without you I would not have moved so far forward in my personal growth on every level. You ladies have left an eternal footprint. We were destined to meet.

Priya, Shanti and Shona: ladies, thank you for all your kindness always.

A special acknowledgement to the 'young ladies': first of all, 'Mathilda marshmallow' for being living proof of being capable of performing a full press-up when you use the strength and power of your mind. 'Lara' for being my youngest fan (at the age of three). I was more popular than Peppa Pig and have adopted the name 'Lala'. Not forgetting 'Layla' who is purely a lovely-natured angel.

To my grandma who is the love of my life, you have taught me pure love just by *being* and leading by example. I love you more than anything imaginable.

Thank you mum for everything you have given me. I love you.

Thank you for always being there for me when I needed you Aunt Janice and to the rest of my kind-hearted family: my Uncle Farhad, Allan, Stuart, Stacy, Phillip, Christopher, Nat and Roger.

Finally, a big heartfelt thank you for all those amazing people whose paths I have crossed on my self-transformational journey.

"The only person who is responsible for mastering our mind, body and soul is ourself"

Lisa Danielle Dominica Smith

# Contents

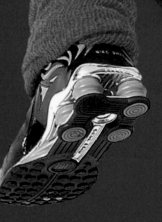

# Contents (continued)

# Introduction

**This book is about fitness of the mind, fitness of the body and fitness of the soul. My aim is to help you transform and grow on every level.**

Many people have asked me how I have managed to sustain my youth and body shape for almost 20 years. My chronological age has never defined me. In fact, in the last seven years of my life, there has been a huge influx of energetic changes internally and externally. This has shifted a great deal of negative emotion which has been replaced by positivity. This feeling has transmitted itself in all of my being, and has drawn comments from friends questioning how I manage to maintain a real sense of peace and calmness within me.

The difference is immeasurable. I feel I have bundles more energy compared to when I was in my twenties. My body is fitter and stronger too. I look aesthetically better. I can even eat more without putting on the weight, even though I was exercising much more in my twenties and early thirties (doing double the exercise I do now). I feel that at 40, as long as I focus my attention, energy and mind, I have an abundance of energy and I can achieve anything I want. I have discovered the infinite power of the mind. I know my search will hopefully lead to an even bigger path of mind and body expansion and perhaps I will be writing *Fabulous Fitness at 50* one day.

It is only now that I realise I have been able to achieve anything I want through the practice of a disciplined mind. It is only in the latter years of my career that I have had the opportunity and privilege to be exposed to this type of thinking through sheer yearning and practise. I now recognise that fitness starts on the inside and real strength originates from the mind.

In this book, I would like to share my experience and knowledge with you.

My intention is to help you develop mentally, evolve spiritually and get stronger physically.

# Ladan's 10 power tools to achieve success of the mind and body, and how to maintain it:

**1** Catch your thoughts and reframe them so you can train the mind to think positively

**2** Reprogram the subconscious mind

**3** Positive affirmations

**4** Law of attraction

**5** Visualisation

**6** Yoga

**7** Breathing techniques

**8** Meditation

**9** Physical exercise

**10** Healthy eating and nutrition

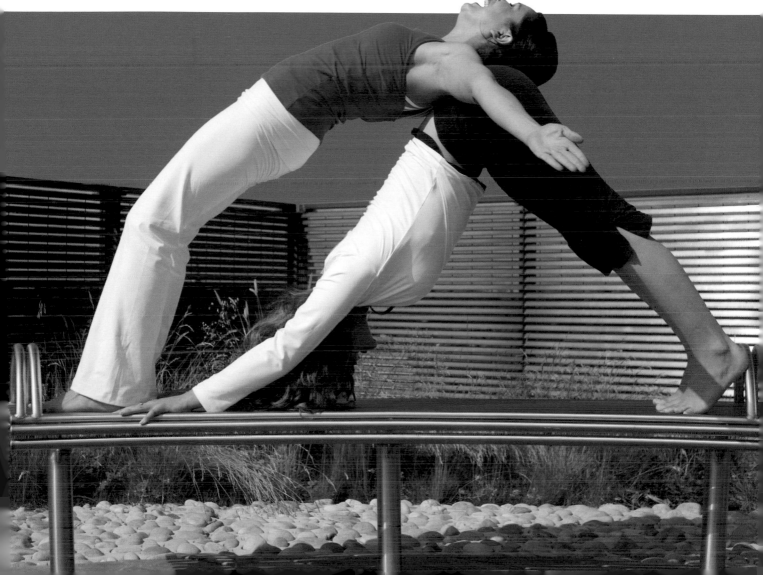

# What is fitness to you?

What's the first thing that pops into your mind when someone mentions the word fitness to you? Does your memory flash back to the days when you were exhausting your body on that treadmill in the hope of stepping off it like a supermodel goddess after the first session? Or, how about when your trainer came round and worked your arms so hard that when you brushed your teeth the next morning the toothbrush had to be placed on the shelf horizontally facing you, while you moved your head from side to side so you could clean your teeth because your arms were off-duty that day? What about the time you wanted to change your body shape three weeks before a holiday, with the hope of dropping four sizes? Yes, in three weeks, and you had owned that body for over 20 years! Hmm, sound all too familiar?

Well, I don't have a magic wand and recipe to get quick, fast, sharp results in 0.1 seconds. However, what I do have is a methodology, using 10 powerful tools that you can apply as an approach to transforming your life. I will teach you how to train your mind to give you the ability to live your life magically. When I say that, I mean we are going to start this journey from the inside out. And it will be a journey that will not be for the moment, but a new lifestyle.

If you haven't guessed by now, I am talking about fitness of the mind, which once you have mastered it, the rest will fall into place and lead to fitness of the physical body. This is the way you are going to sustain longevity and, more importantly, keep the body of your dreams.

So, I hope you're ready to embark upon our mission.

# The mind

Our mind is a huge mass of consciousness. It is a transmitter and receiver of energy. The mind is vast. The mind is so powerful that it is our driving force in life and how we choose to live it. If you can discipline the mind by exercising it every day, just as you would the physical body, then you can change your way of thinking in the same way that you can change the shape of your body when working out. You could even compare it to when you participate in cardio-vascular exercise in order to make the heart (which is a muscle in itself) stronger. This will decrease the resting heart rate meaning that your heart has to beat less beats per minute to pump the blood and oxygen around the body efficiently, hence less wear and tear on the heart: helping you to live longer.

It's the same with your mind, it is just like a muscle that grows and gets stronger. The way to learn to make the mind strong and gain control of your thoughts is by reprogramming it. The aim is to break old habits and not entertain unwanted negative thought patterns.

At first it may seem like you're going backwards, but as your sense of awareness becomes greater you will find that catching your thoughts will help you identify how many times we think with a negative thinking pattern. It may not make you feel great at the beginning of your self-realisation, but once you have gone past this stage and cleansed the old ways of thinking from your mind, you will have a new, positive, fresh outlook at how you view life and other people.

At first, just like when you turn on an old tap which hasn't been in use for years, all the murky water will come out with a pungent odour but finally, after you run it for a while, you will see pure crystal clear water.

Eventually, your new way of thinking will gain momentum in your mind and be the best detox work-out.

Just as we have the conscious and subconscious mind, I believe that we have the option to connect to what I call either 'the higher mind' or 'the instinctive mind'.

# The higher mind

The higher mind is ultimately the vessel in which we are aiming to live, be and think. This is like connecting to a higher part of ourselves where we feel as though we are almost being guided by a higher vibrational force of energy that is bigger than us and carries us if we allow ourselves to surrender to it. If we have the ability and practice to understand how to tap into this higher source, then most of the challenges and blockages which we face in our daily lives will be dealt with in a much easier and less problematic way. For example, to achieve the body of your dreams and keep it will no longer be such a task, but a joy and a chosen way of wanting to live because of how good you feel in your mind.

A fantastic metaphor for always being connected to the higher mind is 'the sky is always blue'. Cast your mind back to when you were flying above the clouds in an aeroplane and all you could see was a stunning, bright blue sky. Then look down at the clouds below you. Even if there is a storm going on in those dark clouds or the weather is thunderous and grey, for you, it really doesn't matter because where you're living in the mind 'the sky is always blue'. This is where I would like to aim to help you to live, in that higher-minded space, so no matter what comes your way in the future you are not going to let it ruin your wonderful serene space that you have chosen to tap into. At the end of the day you have that choice. You can choose to allow one person or event to pollute your mind and

ruin your whole mood. It really is up to you. Do you want it to bring you down or do you accept that it is what it is and trust that it will work out in the way it is meant to?

Surrender to that higher mind and by letting go, that feeling will naturally dissipate and it will be dealt with in a much calmer state.

Later, I will be teaching you some meditation techniques and mind exercises to help you master your mind. It is again a practice which will be more successful depending on how much effort you invest. If you train your body frequently in the gym by using different styles of work-outs and cross training it will look better, the same rule applies to exercising the mind.

Think about how it feels when you take up a new fitness activity. At first your motor coordination is really being challenged and your flexibility is being stretched to the limit. Your muscles ache so much that you can't possibly imagine it ever getting any easier. Then you start to practise regularly and your body gets stronger. Then you start notching up the intensity, frequency and perhaps double up the weights and repetitions. You can do exactly the same with your mind. As everything originates from here, the root connection of how you live your life, then why not start to exercise the mind and learn how to gain mastery of it? This of course leads you to gain control of your whole life.

# The instinctive mind (relating to the physical body)

The instinctive mind is connected to eating, sleeping and procreation. You could say that it is the mind which is more associated with the animalistic way of being. As humans, if we are only functioning in this mind space, I would say we are only living in survival mode and hardly using any of our mind's capacity. It's widely believed we are only using a limited amount of our minds and from personal experience I would say that the mind has much more infinite potential (see my

biography on page 122 for real-life examples of this). Not to explore and tap into the mind's unlimited possibilities would be merely living an existence as opposed to living life to the fullest and the best of our ability. There are periods in our life due to unforeseen circumstances where we just about cope. In these periods we can only maintain living our life in this instinctive space.

Unfortunately, living with emotional/clinical disorders and other forms of psychological or physiological issues can really drag us down.

We can choose to give in and continue living like this on a dead-end slope, or we can have the courage to pick ourselves up and use all the possible resources available to us.

If you want to help yourself and do good to others and contribute to the world, the universe will always be there to help you. You simply have to ask for it and trust and believe that you deserve to receive it.

# The conscious and subconscious mind

## The conscious mind

Our conscious mind is connected to the real world we live in, which means whatever we have created as our own personal reality. Every individual has their own ways of understanding things and how they process information and behave in certain situations.

The conscious mind governs everything we do with awareness. It uses logic and rational thinking.

It is about all the thoughts you are conscious of, the thoughts which will direct and inform you, and the thoughts which control how you must be.

Ultimately, it is the belief in your own conscious mind which will bring about the results on how you live your life.

## The subconscious mind

It is the subconscious mind that controls our behaviour and emotions most of the time. Believe it or not, the core of your feelings originates from the subconscious and manifests into the conscious.

The subconscious mind is connected to all our feelings and experiences of the past. This of course continues to influence us in our daily lives even though we may not be aware of it. Old patterns, habits and ways of thinking are all part of the stored information in our subconscious. You use the subconscious for all that you have learned without thinking. The subconscious mind works and learns by repetition.

When you are learning something new, for example, a new fitness routine or training programme, you are using the conscious mind. However, once you have grasped the routine, you then pass this information to the subconscious mind. Just as you would download and store information on a computer, you could call the subconscious mind your hard drive. Let's say you tried to lose weight and started an exercise regime in the past and the results were not successful. When it came to shifting the last few pounds it became impossible, which possibly made you very despondent and caused you to give in. You then punish yourself a) for giving up and b) because of the guilt and defeat. These feelings about this event will be stored in your subconscious. Then the next time you try dieting and weight loss, instead of having a whole new fresh approach to the idea that you will reach your goal successfully, in your subconscious somewhere you will still be holding onto the old feelings in relation to your past experience, causing you to feel the same emotions, thus creating a blockage. Your conscious mind knows how to rationalise this, however, the subconscious is telling it something different.

I'm only brushing the surface here with the two dynamic mind sets which are fascinating subjects. However, the most important thing to remember is that the subconscious mind believes everything you tell it. It does not argue with you, it takes orders from the conscious. If you decide to look at yourself in the mirror and tell yourself 'I feel fat' and keep thinking exactly that, well guess what? Your subconscious is going to believe you. If you look at yourself and say 'I feel fantastic', then the same philosophy applies, you will feel fantastic and others around you will pick up on that vibe.

In this book, we are going to learn some techniques for reprogramming the subconscious mind by catching your thoughts and changing them around. It is almost like teaching yourself a new language. The magic of this is that you have to be conscious and really concentrate on staying present at first. Eventually, like the losing weight metaphor, it will sink into your subconscious and your natural way of thinking without any effort will only be positive. This is the first step to learning how to work out and exercise your mind. Remember fitness starts from the inside out, because the only way out is by going in.

> *The conscious mind may be compared to a fountain playing in the sun and falling back into the great subterranean post of subconscious from which it rises.*
>
> Sigmund Freud

# Our thoughts

### What are thoughts?

Our thoughts are a vibration of energy. While light travels at the rate of approximately 186,282 miles per second, our thoughts virtually travel in no time. The velocity of thought is unimaginable. It is a dynamic force, if you go with the notion that every thought you send out is a vibration which never perishes.

As I have already mentioned, our mind is a transmitter and receiver of energy. As our thoughts are made up of energy, a great analogy to understand and recognise the sheer power of the consequences of how your thoughts affect yourself and others is: if you have a bad thought about someone, not only are you sending them negative vibes, you are also toxicating yourself and contaminating the mental atmosphere. What I mean by the latter is that your thoughts travel out by giving rise to vibration into the universe. That thought energy travels in all directions into the cosmic consciousness. It will cross the mind of that person who you have had that thought about. Have you ever noticed that when you have been thinking about someone in particular they suddenly call you for no apparent reason after so many years? Well what do you think this means? This is a clear sign that we have so much more power in our thinking than we give credit to.

I'd like you to try this as an exercise, think of somebody with whom you would like to resume contact again and see how quickly you will hear from this person.

Thoughts are like a boomerang, whatever you send out, guaranteed (good or bad), will come back.

We are made up of our thoughts, that is who we are. Think about it. You have a thought or a desire, you act on this thought, this thought becomes a way of being or thinking, therefore this becomes your habit. This way of thinking, or habit, shapes your character and this becomes the way you live your life, the life in which you have created your own destiny by the way you think.

We are the masters and creators of how we live our life and shape our destiny.

### Desire – action – habit – character – destiny

As I have already mentioned, our thoughts make us who we are and mould our lives. In the Swami Sivananda book *Thought Power* it says that we have on average 70,000 thoughts a day, and remember, this is simply an average quote. It is probably much higher for the overloaded, anxious-minded individual. Now how much control do you think you have over these thoughts? Are you aware that you can catch your thoughts? We have the ability to completely switch them around. In an ideal world we would like to be programmed to always think in a positive way.

Why is it that some people have the ability and self-discipline to achieve and maintain their ideal body? Yet for others it

is an ongoing struggle, one which they end up losing. What have the high achievers got that the others lack? Well, we are all humans functioning with the same gifts and abilities therefore we are all able to succeed in exactly the same way. I will be teaching you visualisation techniques and meditation to aid in making the mind stronger.

# Learn how to discipline and master your mind

Let us begin to train our minds by initially observing thought patterns. I want us to start with an exercise of simply catching your thoughts. Now, our awareness at the beginning has to be turned up to the highest volume. Remember, we are now dealing with the conscious mind. Some of you may be very surprised with what comes up for you with this exercise. Perhaps you were not aware that you have literally always thought like this. I want you to go and stand by a mirror,

ideally full length. Take a good look at yourself and while you're doing this let your thoughts come up and just witness how many of these thoughts are negative and how many positive.

What is your mind saying to you? Who else came into your mind? Were you being nice about yourself or anyone else who popped into your mind?

**Write a list of all your thoughts, positive and negative:**

_____

_____

_____

_____

_____

_____

_____

_____

Stay with this exercise for the next few days and be a witness to what comes up. I think it is a good idea to write down all the thoughts you are hearing about yourself. You don't have to do this just by standing in front of the mirror. Start to be what I call on 'thought duty' all the time, especially when you are carrying out other tasks. This will really make you live consciously and raise your sense of awareness to the voices and endless chitter-chatter in your head.

> This week I'm going to be a bouncer on 'thought duty'. I will stand at the gate of my mind watching closely the entering thoughts. Negative thoughts: be warned, you are not on the list! You will be exterminated instantly. I only entertain and welcome positive, sublime thoughts. We all have the ability to be the avatars of our thoughts…

After you have practised this exercise for a while and taken a mental note of your thought patterns by being the observer, I'd like you now to treat your mind as though it is the most breathtaking, lush green garden. Imagine this garden has beautiful flowers. In fact, the flowers are so amazing to look at that even our conditioned eyes have now been witness to see colours they never knew existed. What I'd like you to imagine is that this incredible garden is your mind. Now put some gates in front of this garden and keep it protected and guarded. Next, I would like you to imagine that every single negative thought you have is a weed. There is no room for weeds to spoil this glorious place and if they start to pop up, they will have to be removed (filtered out) instantly.

This is a great metaphor to get you started in catching your thoughts and stop your mind and body absorbing them. You can also create your own analogy of how you want to protect and guard your mind against harmful, wreckless thoughts.

When you have any thought, it is conveyed into every single cell in your body. Once this transmits, your body will physiologically be affected by whatever it is you have been thinking about. Think about it, you are asked to do something which is really going to challenge you and put you way out of your comfort zone. What is the first thing which pops into your mind? Fear? Sound familiar? What happens next, your heartbeat goes up because your breathing pattern changes to shallow breathing. This is due to the fact that there is an intimate connection between thinking and respiration, and also between the mind and the breath. The shallow breath and fearful thought starts to affect the nervous system and your digestive system. This of course affects your respiratory system which eventually affects the adrenals which have to secrete more cortisol, the hormone produced to control stress in the body when it is under the fight or flight state. This will have a knock-on effect on your endocrine system and all the hormones go out of sync with one another. All this with one negative thought connected to fear. Wow, that is how much power one single negative thought can have.

Now remember, this works both ways and in my personal opinion, when we entertain positive thoughts, the outcome is even more amplified on the physical body than anything with negative form. Positivity always outweighs negativity. I will explain how this works. Imagine walking into a dark room. It is so dark that even your eyes cannot really get used to it. What do you do so you can see? Obviously you light a match or a candle and there you have light. Now let's assume we are in a bright, light room. How can you make that room so dark, that you can't even see anything? That explains the sheer power of positivity. This is a grand effective law of nature, just as darkness cannot stand before the sun.

If you find that some days your thoughts are negative and making you feel out of control, I suggest another exercise. As soon as you hear something which doesn't resonate with you positively, change the thought straight away. Let us go back to that voice saying, 'I feel fat, I feel ugly'. The second you hear that, catch it and reframe that thought. Change it by replacing it immediately and say, 'I love my body and I feel beautiful'. Vocalise it out loud to the negative voice and tell it 'I don't believe you!'. Speak to it and say 'go away, your words are not welcome here'. Physically tell that thought that you want nothing to do with it. You will be very surprised by how empowering this feels. You literally disassociate yourself with these thought forms by addressing 'that's not me', and 'these are external words which don't belong to me'.

We cannot always be on guard to control our thoughts, however with practise we have the ability to control our words and with repetition we can master the thoughts of the subconscious.

Start by changing one negative thought at a time. Usually it is the first one which pops into your head that has a knock-on domino effect on all the other thoughts which arise from the original source. Stop it as soon as you hear it. For example, when you hear 'I feel fat, I feel ugly', from there on you will hear all other related thoughts like, 'well even my stomach looks bloated and disgusting', which loads onto 'my face is so spotty and ugly' and the list goes on and on.

Remember as I have already mentioned, the subconscious believes everything you tell it. The aim of these exercises is to reprogram this part of your mind and train it to only entertain sublime thoughts. If you keep feeding positive thoughts to your mind, eventually, your mind will only function in this empowered way. Thoughts gain strength and power through repetition. Just as the same birds of a feather flock together, collective, positive thoughts will start to breed forever.

Always try to cultivate this way of thinking and get rid of old habitual thought patterns about yourself and others. Feed your mind only with nourished thoughts just as you would your physical body if you were on an organic wholesome eating plan. You will start to see a huge energetic shift within yourself and even notice the difference of how people are magnetically drawn towards your radiating, infectious energy.

We are always talking about inhaling industrial toxic chemicals or eating foods which are so mass manufactured that all the goodness is destroyed, leaving no nutritious value in the product for us. Well what do you think negative thoughts are? They are the worst form of contamination for your mind and body.

# Positive versus negative

## Positive thoughts

Have you ever been in the presence of positive people and realised how inspired and motivated you felt in their company?

A person who is connected to a higher vibrational realm, or their higher self, emanates positivity. The word 'emanates' derives from the latin word emanare which means 'flowing from'. Positive thoughts arise from an uplifted cheerful disposition. Positive thoughts are thoughts of unlimited potential which will generate abundance and expand our awareness in aiding us to overcome difficulty. Always remember, positivity breeds positivity.

## Negative thoughts

As you already know we have an unbelievable volume of thoughts going through our minds each and every second. Unfortunately, a high ratio of these thoughts harbour negativity. Just as you have been in the presence of positive people and felt the effects, the same applies for being around negative people. If you are with a person who is consumed with negativity, this can leave you feeling tired and deflated. Unless your mind is strong and stable, it is inevitable that you can absorb the dark under-toned vibrations. This is why it is vital for us to enrich and empower our minds with pure thoughts. We do not want to buy into a negative person's limiting belief system.

Negative thoughts are characterised by feelings of hatred, spite, jealousy and anger, to name a few. These thoughts are often supported by anxiety, manipulation, discrimination and judgement. Negative thoughts restrict and confine your sense of self and self-belief if we choose to believe them. Practise and learn to recognise fearful thoughts which debilitate you. This fearful state drives the life force out of us, creating blockages and stopping us evolving positively. This will assist us in our process of overcoming negative thought patterns.

If we have had negative past experiences, which I am sure we all have, this will be remembered through the subconscious.

As you know this information will be downloaded on the template of our subconscious and played to us repetitively unless we have the strength and courage to change it. The process in which all these bad habits will dissolve are through the practice of reprogramming your way of thinking.

Many of our past experiences didn't work out in the way we might have hoped they would. This can leave you feeling unfulfilled. Don't allow yourself to wallow in a victim state and drown in the sea of darkness, where every single cell in your body will be sapped dry of energy. Start to let go of negative thinking patterns which have been sabotaging your mind with limiting beliefs. Now is the time to adopt a powerful thinking technique and manifest living a life of positive abundance by being the architect of your articulate thoughts.

There is one positive thing about having a negative thought. If you acknowledge the negative immediately, this will allow you to replace it with a positive one. Having negative thoughts makes you harness only positive thoughts if you choose to live with awareness.

> *Negative folks need positive strokes.*
>
> Unknown

# Positive thinking and living

Start to see problems you face as an opportunity to grow and shape your life. Look for the seed of something better when life feels like a struggle. Remember, train your mind to see and trust that experiencing misfortune will have a positive outcome. Practise looking at the bigger picture and have faith that this has happened for a reason in order for you to grow and learn a lesson from. It may not seem like a learning curve for you at the time. However, eventually as events in your life unfold you will think 'aha, I understand now'.

Maybe in the past you have tried and explored many different ways to diet and lose weight and just when you felt like you were heading on the right track, some family situation evolved. Or perhaps your boss was giving you endless amounts of work which prevented you from going to the gym as frequently as you had hoped. Instead of thinking this was going to be an impossible task and wanting to give up instantly, use this as an opportunity to cultivate an attitude to ask yourself 'What is there to learn from this?'

There is a meaning to be had from every moment in tremendous suffering. Perhaps this situation has taught you to manage your time better and to be even more conscientious in order to reach your goal.

I know for a fact, the more we do, the more we realise we can do. Maybe you haven't had the time to perform all your exercises in the gym and feel upset with yourself for not doing this. How about focusing on all the exercises you did complete? What if your boss has sacked you and you feel like a failure. Stay optimistic and remind yourself that this was the end of a chapter of your life and, even though you are sad, be excited about the prospect of the next stage of your life. Perhaps this would be a fantastic opportunity to start to invest more time in your health in the interim while looking for a new job. We have to constantly remind ourselves to start investing in our health now, regardless of the obstacles we are up against. This will change your whole outlook and make the mind stronger. Remember fitness starts in the mind.

This new way of mind intervention will give you the self-realisation that the grass is not greener on the other side; in fact you are already standing on the greenest grass.

This will help boost your confidence and promote self-esteem and self-belief. Keep on believing in yourself.

---

*Believers are achievers who always receive what they perceive.*

Ladan Soltani

---

By now you are aware that fostering positive wholesome thoughts can transform the outlook of a person. Your thoughts can change your life and let you live the lifestyle that you have always dreamed of. Get rid of all the useless information which has accumulated and has stored in the brain taking up mind space. Learn to un-mind the mind and make room for those divine thoughts to come flowing in. Never underestimate the sheer velocity of your thoughts.

In the early stages of learning to reprogram your mind and control your thoughts, you will experience great challenges. I call these challenges 'growing pains'. Just as when you start a new fitness regime you discover that within those first few weeks your poor body is literally aching in pain. This is the time that the muscles are repairing themselves in order to grow and get stronger. This same rule applies to your thought practice.

At first you will notice that the negative thoughts refuse to be shunned out of your mind. They will start a war with your positive mind and demand that they remain as inhabitants and try to take full ownership of the space in which they breed. They will refuse to leave and may even take hostages. They will try every single trick in the book to take up sole residency in your mind. However, we know that positivity outweighs negativity and this will encourage you to be even more determined and motivated to complete your task.

Just as you start seeing small changes in your physical body from all the exercises, you will witness refreshing ways of how your mind is starting to untangle itself away from the negative thoughts. Eventually, through practice, introspection and vigilance you will only be attracted towards the positive thoughts.

Once you start to follow the path of positive thinking, you will want to expand and remain in the higher mind realm. My recommendation is that you make it a goal to hang around with like-minded people. Stay focused and concentrate your efforts on stretching your mind's capacity by reading inspiring books or taking courses. It is exactly like training your body. Once you start to see a change in your body, you need to maintain it and cross train it further to take the results to the next level.

You will have days when you feel out of control and get ruled by negative, fearful thoughts. Remember to have compassion and cultivate kindness to yourself as this is the best vitamin for your mind. Sometimes we have to accept these feelings and sit with them. It may not feel comfortable at first, in fact, accepting these thoughts and feelings until they dissolve resembles a 'cold turkey' state. Patience is key. Let these moments pass by. Accept how you feel as fighting against it will only block the situation furthermore.

When you feel like your thought pattern is starting to dip downhill, I suggest the following exercise:

Make a list of 20 things that you have that you are grateful for. Being grateful and living in gratitude enriches your mind. You may feel that 20 is quite a significant amount, however, once you start to write you will be really surprised at the result. In fact, it is more realistic that the number doubles for you.

23

**A list of things which I am grateful for:**

1

2

3

4

5

6

7

8

9

10

11

12

13

14

15

16

17

18

19

20

Good. Now read this and sit with the feelings you gain from doing this. Feel the waves of joy and happiness and appreciate what you are experiencing.

Once you start to live and evolve in a positive space, naturally, you will start to attract like-minded people into your life. Your personality will radiate magnetism and people will gravitate towards you. People will seek you out requesting your recipe for staying so focused and positive.

I know two wonderful stories which clearly demonstrate the idea that who we invite into our lives represents a mirror image of ourselves.

Once upon a time, there was a beautiful princess. One day, she decided to go for a walk into a huge hall of mirrors in the palace. When she got there and took a look in the mirrors, she noticed a really beautiful princess staring back at her. This brought up a lot of rage and jealousy. How can she be more beautiful than me? The more she thought about it, the more angry she got, the more angry she got, the more the other princesses in the other mirrors got angry. This made her

blood pressure go up so high that she was absolutely fuming. Suddenly, she had a heart attack!

Or, once upon a time, there was a beautiful princess. One day, she decided to go for a walk into a huge hall of mirrors in the palace. When she got there and took a look in the mirrors, she noticed a really beautiful princess staring back at her. When she saw her, she smiled. She noticed that when she smiled, all the other princesses in the other mirrors smiled back at her. She was happy that there were so many beautiful princesses in one room. The whole day her heart was filled with joy.

As an experiment, you can go out and smile at ten people and see what happens. Alternatively, if you want to you can look miserable and see what you attract back. You may already know this because if you are reading this book it is with the knowledge that a lot of the content resonates with you. However, actually putting it into practice so that you can own and share that experience is a whole new ball game.

# Positive affirmations

## What are positive affirmations?

Affirmations are assertive, positive words or phrases which help in directing your focus thus enabling you to accomplish all your dreams and passions in life. You can use these powerful statements to conquer your fears which have imprisoned you and prevented you from leading the successful life you deserve to live.

As you know, through repetition of these words, one can reprogram the subconscious mind. If you repeat these daily affirmations on a regular basis and integrate them into your everyday life, just as you regularly brush your teeth, you will notice the difference in your sense of self-belief and confidence.

When you first start repeating your affirmations, the subconscious mind may react with resistance.

If you feel challenged and move towards staying with the subconscious mind's perceived inner truth, you will start to feel a strong negative feeling within you. This means it will take a little longer to work. However, equally if you feel a sense of well-being, your mind is naturally responding to something it believes to be true. When you feel this emotion, you know your affirmations are working.

The more determined you are in making these changes and the more willing to accept change and let go of your past way of thinking, the sooner and more effectively these affirmations will work for you. The time frame is down to you and how quickly you are ready to adapt to change, as opposed to how long it will take in order for it to work.

I will demonstrate a sample of positive affirmations which you can use for yourself. If you choose to create your own, be specific about what you want. Once you have thought of them, repeat them daily with conviction. Mean what you say and be passionate. When you are saying the 'feel good' affirmations make a mental note of how you are feeling. If you're vocalising an affirmation about your body, visualise your lean, svelte, toned body as you're saying it.

**Examples of positive affirmations:**

▸ 'Every day in every way, I love myself more and more'
▸ 'Today I have been blessed to begin an inner journey that will last the rest of my life'
▸ 'I love how I look'
▸ 'Each and every day, I'm getting thinner and fitter'
▸ 'I love my life'
▸ 'I feel fantastic'
▸ 'I love feeling fit'
▸ 'Keeping fit is effortless'
▸ 'When I honour myself, I have more compassion'
▸ 'I always aspire higher'
▸ 'I like myself'
▸ 'I believe and achieve anything I want'
▸ 'I enjoy feeling healthy'
▸ 'I am filled with energy and vitality'
▸ 'I have bundles of energy'
▸ 'I feel ready to accept change in my life'
▸ 'I feel a sense of peace and joy'
▸ 'My thoughts are pure and positive'
▸ 'I am a vessel of positive energy'
▸ 'I channel my thoughts positively'
▸ 'I believe in myself'
▸ 'Hot chips? No thanks, I love my hot hips'
▸ 'Good things come to me'
▸ 'I am living in a blissful space'
▸ 'I can eat delicious food and keep my slender figure'
▸ 'When I help myself, the universe helps me more'
▸ 'I have gratitude for the wonderful things in my life'
▸ 'I deserve to live a happy, fulfilling life'

I have a simple metaphor to share with you. I would like you to try this so you can understand and feel how powerful affirmations are:

Pick up a set of weights. They don't have to be heavy. (Use a water bottle if you don't have weights).

Lift both weights laterally to each side so your arms come up in line with your chest and your palms are facing downwards. Keep the weights there for about ten seconds. Now relax your arms and close your eyes. Tell yourself that you are really weak and that you have no energy left to lift the weights. Now do exactly that, if you can lift the weights up to where they were before and keep repeating this like an affirmation. 'I am weak, I have no strength, I have no energy' How does it feel? Could you keep the weights up there without a struggle? Now relax your arms and close your eyes. I want you to tell yourself that you are the strongest person in the world. Lift the weights up to the desired position and keep repeating this affirmation adding you have bundles of energy. How does it feel? This is a simple analogy and living proof of the power of affirmation.

# Other people's negative affirmations

When you are in the company of negative people who hold you back with their uninspiring words, you will find being in this space uncomfortable, especially if you have been chanting your positive affirmations.

I have a story to share which is an excellent example of why you should not listen and be discouraged by other people's negative words.

Once upon a time, there was a bunch of monkeys who wanted to enter a running competition to climb a huge tower. On the day of the race everyone was telling them it was impossible. As the race was about to begin, the crowd of people gathered to the top of the tower. One by one the monkeys started to climb up the tower and as they were climbing, the crowd was calling down with messages like 'Stop now or you will injure yourself!', 'You monkeys are mad, you will never make it!', 'Dream on if you want to make it to the top!'

As the monkeys started to hear these messages, slowly one by one they became discouraged and started to drop out. The crowd got louder with their applause of negative words. Eventually most of the monkeys started to give up for various reasons. 'Maybe they're right,' said one monkey to another, 'perhaps we are over ambitious that we can make it.'

The race came to an end and only one monkey managed to climb the whole tower with a huge smile on his face. When he got to the finish line all the other monkeys were intrigued at how this other monkey managed to climb the tower. When they spoke to him they realised he was deaf.

The moral of this story goes for any negative external influences we have in our life. When someone is telling you that your dream is impossible, catch their sentence as you would a negative thought and reframe it. Amend the statement and turn it around and thank them for encouraging you to accomplish your mission even more.

# Super-empowered affirmations

To enhance the power of these affirmations, write them down on sticky notes and stick them everywhere. Put them on your fridge, especially if you want to lose weight and each time you want to go in the fridge you have to pass through your affirmation as a reminder.

Stand in front of the mirror and say it out loud. Words are very powerful and sound vibrates out into the universe. Look at yourself as you are saying this and amplify the magnification of your words. Own your words and let them become your own sacred mantra.

You can also make a song out of your affirmations. Or perhaps create a rhyme out of your affirmations so you can always remember them. Keep your affirmations short and to the point and start your day with a daily routine. As soon as you wake up start your day in a positive way.

Through constant repetition of these daily affirmations, without effort, you will subconsciously be saying them in your head. This will totally transform your mind and help create what you have always envisioned to have in your life.

If you want to look fabulous and feel fantastic, let these affirmations be your free supplements which complement your healthy eating plan and your exercise regime.

Make a list of all your affirmations on the following page and start to validate and manifest them. Remember to say them all in the present tense.

**List of affirmations:**

# The law of attraction

### What is the law of attraction?

The law of attraction is about how we create our own reality and manifest the life we wish to live. We create our reality by focusing our attention onto the desired goal. Most people, without being aware, will put their energy and thought power into exactly what they don't want, thus resulting in an outcome of getting exactly what they don't want as they have created that as their reality.

Instead, you need to focus on more of what you do want and less of what you don't want. This is the way to live your life by the 'law of attraction philosophy'.

Have you noticed that people who always complain of being sick and that they have a miserable life in fact live that lifestyle? Yet on the other side of the coin, people who talk about prosperity and having a lavish appetite and zest for life get to live like kings. In fact, the people who live by the latter wouldn't even consider or comprehend how to live any other way because they live by the law of attraction naturally.

It is such an empowered way to live that any negativity implemented into the space probably wouldn't stand a chance to survive. It is highly likely the thought would instantly be crushed by the positive mental vibration.

### How does the law of attraction work?

As you are well aware, we don't need to study physics to understand how gravity works. We all know about 'Newton's law' as in what goes up, must come down. Simply throwing a ball in the air demonstrates that. Well the same rule applies for the law of attraction. As you know by now, 'your thoughts become things' hence the famous saying 'as you think, so you become'.

Thought governs our lives and that which you desire is simply a thought away. Well, the law of attraction is an immutable law as predictable as gravity. You may start with a small thought like a drop in the ocean. This will lead into creating a ripple and potentially it will gain so much momentum that eventually you will cause a current with a tremendous impact.

# The universe

The universe is a mass of consciousness fundamentally filled with information. Everything in the universe is made of energy, including ourselves. This huge vacuum of energy is infinite: it always has and always will be. What can change, however, is our consciousness. We have the potential by using the law of attraction to tap into this vast source of energy and create the life we desire to have.

### Where is this consciousness?

This consciousness lies between the gaps in our thoughts. It is the space of solitude and stillness which connects us to this divine energy.

# The universe loves speed

When you know exactly what you want and have a strong emotion attached to what you desire, the quicker you will receive it because the thought behind your desire has a magnetic frequency. When you want to help yourself, the universe will help you, especially more so when the nature of your thought will impact other people's lives collectively to have a positive effect on them as well as yourself.

# Metaphysics

Metaphysics is what determines the study of the nature of reality, mind and matter. It can constitute a higher reality or the invisible nature behind everything. It is about your life and how you live your life.

# Visualisation

Start by placing a picture in your mind for each thought. Visualise exactly what you want then let it go into the universe without attachment. Treat it like a cosmic order and align yourself with the universe and trust. You must also be open to receive it. Once you have let it go, accept that the universe will bring you what you have manifested and know that you deserve it. All you need to do from here on is feel the feelings of what it is like to have what you have asked for. For example, you want to look a certain way for your summer holiday. Start to visualise how you would like your body to look and sit with how it feels to have it. Close your eyes for a second and visualise your body on the beach and how it feels having it. Hopefully you will feel a tingle or sparkle of energy in your body: that in itself is setting the vibration of the result.

Remember for every action, there is a reaction. You have to be confident in asking for what you want. Ask yourself have you ever asked for help from a higher source bigger than us? Just as you would ask your partner or family for help, ask the universe and start to make small steps, yet think big. Program your destiny like you would a GPS system before a journey in your car.

Through practise of visualisation and positive thoughts you can run towards your fears instead of running away from them. If you embrace them by accepting them, it becomes much easier to let go and be free.

If you want something and allow fear to become an obstacle, the law of attraction cannot bring you your request. Imagine there is a locked door behind which lies your dream and passion yet you are too afraid to open it to find out.

Also, if you are really desperately holding onto something that you badly want, you are actually blocking the energy of inviting your desired outcome. It is like the metaphor of being really constipated. The more you want to release, the more your body holds on and generates tension.

Remember to ask for what you want…

Let it go with no attachment…

Trust you deserve to have it…

Align yourself to receive…

Feel the feelings of having it…

# Visual board

A visual board is a representation of wishes.

You will need some strong paper or cardboard, scissors, glue and magazines or newspaper cuttings.

You make a collage of pictures from magazines or newspapers that contain all the things you would like in your life such as love, health, business, home and well-being. Making a visual board can be fun. It is a fantastic way of knowing exactly how you want your life to be and look. Your personal visual board is only limited by the extent of your own creativity. The great part is that it is very cheap to make and all you really need apart from magazines or newspapers to make your cuttings are your dreams.

Once you have created your board, place it somewhere you can see it everyday. Visual exposure is very important to help it to manifest. To make it work even more, look at it first thing in the morning when you wake up so you can start your day with an illustrated vision of your future. If you look at it last thing at night and sleep on it, these messages will get soaked up into your subconscious and gain intensity while you're asleep.

When I personally created my first vision board two years ago I was unaware of its power. I cut out images from magazines with positive affirmations to go along side it without any expectation of the outcome. To be honest, I wasn't sure if I believed in it. When I completed my board, I actually put it in a pile and forgot about it (not now, my board is now up on my fridge). A few months after I made my board, out of curiosity I looked for it and I could not believe how I had managed to have three things on it which I thought were impossible in such a short space of time. Please don't knock it until you try it. You will be amazed by the outcome and this will only motivate you to keep making them.

Remember when you are making your vision board, surround yourself with the images of who you want to become and just like magic, your life will change and you will gravitate towards the images you have produced for your desired outcome.

# Super-fast results of the law of attraction

When you practice the law of attraction in conjunction with visualisation the fusion of the two becomes very powerful. However, if you want to be even more specific about your goal, choose a time and set a date of when you would want to receive it.

Write a list of all the things you want to receive and give your achieved desires and goals even more power to set them in motion. Once you start to feel the vibration of how it feels when you have reached your goals, you will become a magnet which attracts the desired outcome of what you have manifested. Remember visualise and rehearse your future with every fibre of your being until it becomes your reality.

# Utilising the law of attraction to manifest your ideal body shape and fitness

As we have already mentioned, ultimately to get the desired outcome and create the reality, you have to live it as though you already have it. You have to make it a present living philosophy. When you want to ascertain a certain way of feeling healthy and looking fit, remember to put all your attention and focus into how you want to look and feel and the rest will happen. Learn to accept compliments from others and be kind and compassionate towards yourself.

If you want to keep on being successful in your training and eating plan yet fear lack of self motivation after one month, don't keep telling yourself 'I don't want to plateau and be discouraged', 'I don't want to gain weight again', 'I'm not eating bread' or 'I will never drink again'. These affirmations may seem positive to you, however, you are only giving power to exactly what you don't want. If your focus is to lose weight and that is all you're talking about, then you are really concentrating on the subject of 'weight'. A much healthier affirmation would be 'I live thin', 'I feel thin', 'I deserve this slender figure' or 'I have bundles of energy and vitality'.

Remember the image you portray triggers the subconscious about what it is that you are going to create. One has to trick the mind to create the emotions that send out the vibration which attracts and sends back the result of what you want. If you want to look strong and lean and one of your goals is to lift heavier weights than before, you have to visualise yourself lifting them. Support this image with a relevant affirmation, such as 'I am the strongest person in the world'. If you want to run a race and be first, close your eyes and visualise yourself crossing the line first and hear the roaring cheer of the crowd and your supporters.

Tests have proved that if you feed patients with subliminal messages by rewiring the brain and painting pictures of what you want to look like, concentrating all your focus and energy into this will set the vibes in motion to come into fruition. Not only will you get the physically fit body you wished for but you will keep dropping the pounds and chances are you are more likely to keep it off in the long term.

# Playing the game of believing your future exists in the present

This is an interesting game to play on your own, or to share collectively in a group if you want to gain greater momentum.

Think of something you would love to have in your life. Imagine you have already achieved it. Now talk about it as if it has happened.

Let's take the example that perhaps you would love to qualify to become a fitness trainer and help others with your knowledge and expertise. First you start out by saying loudly to your friends, to the group or in the mirror, 'I remember the day when I completed my fitness training course and passed

with top results. Then I applied for a job at an exclusive health club who only take on the best teachers. When I got the job I was so happy and excited about having the opportunity to help so many people that I got rewarded as the best newcomer. I love working in this heath club, etc.'

By doing this you are simply affirming your future and creating the feelings which go with the desired outcome.

When you try this yourself, you will feel such a high and your mood will instantly feel lifted and elevated.

If you were not sure how to create the feelings of your desired outcome to activate the law of attraction, then this is a great way to start doing it.

Start by making your goals into realities. Cover every aspect of your life. Make a list by writing down all your future goals here as if you have already achieved them.

**A list of my future goals:**

The tools I have provided for you in this section are there to be utilised. They will not change anything in your life if you don't start to apply them. Make sure your tools don't live in your tool box and stay shiny, clean and unlikely to come out in case they get dirty. In a few months your tools should have accumulated a few chips and dents or perhaps be in need of tiny repairs. If this is the case, then you have done a great job in applying them.

This information is to help you discover your full inner potential by getting to know the teacher/guru within yourself. I can help inspire you with my words, however, the person who has the wisdom to seek solely for the infinite answers, recognises that all the answers lie within themselves...

# Chapter 2
# Yoga and Meditation

# What is yoga?

Yoga is an ancient eastern spiritual practice that uses metaphysical philosophy and postures, that dates back more than 5000 years. This time-honoured tradition has explored every dimension of life and being. It is a scientific system of total development of the physical, mental and spiritual.

Yoga caters universally. Whether you are a professional, academic, or unwaged, mother, senior or child, the yogic way can be incorporated and integrated into your life.

The Sanskrit word (ancient language of India) yug means 'yoke' or 'to join', which is where the name yoga derives from. Essentially, it means that we as human beings are all connected to one another as part of the cosmos. The whole concept behind the yoga theory is that we understand our connection and union with one another and to the 'absolute whole'. Its purpose is to aid us to live more consciously and learn to banish ignorance.

Yoga is the path to liberation and enlightenment through the practice and understanding of how to let go of material desires and free the spirit. It is a true representation of 'simple living' yet 'high thinking'. It is a valuable resource for those who seek to find the ultimate truth within themselves and live their daily life as a 'yogi'. In the west, yoga is identified by its postures and attaining a lean and toned body. While these are some of the benefits, there are many other branches associated with yoga.

# The four branches of yoga

## Raja (or Ashtanga) Yoga

The fundamental of Raja Yoga is the correlation of the mind with balancing emotions. It is not unusual to classify Raja Yoga as the 'king of yogas' because of its scientific approach. The techniques used in this type of yoga aim to achieve higher states of being and consciousness.

Raja Yoga has eight limbs (aspects) which were compiled by Patanjali Maharishi (a well-known Sage) in the yoga sutras (Hindu scripture).

The practice of Raja Yoga is the path of systematic analysis and mind control. These eight steps are a series of disciplines which the 'yogi' practices to purify and cleanse the body and mind in order to attain enlightenment. It is also known as Ashtanga Yoga. Here are the Sanskrit terms with their meanings:

▶ **Yamas** *restraints*
▶ **Niyamas** *observances*
▶ **Asanas** *postures*
▶ **Pranayama** *breathing*
▶ **Pratyahara** *internalising the senses*
▶ **Dharana** *concentration*
▶ **Dhyana** *meditation*
▶ **Samadhi** *supreme consciousness*

### *Yamas and niyamas*

Within the yamas and niyamas you have the following five moral character and ethical conducts or restraints. The yamas focus on destroying the lower nature and the niyamas on adopting a positive attitude and qualities.

### Yamas

*Ahimsa* – non-violence and abstaining from causing harm to others

*Satya* – honesty and being sincere with your words

*Brahmacharya* – sublimination of the sexual energy

*Asteya* – non-possessiveness and not stealing

*Aparigraha* – living in moderation

**Niyamas**

*Saucha* – living purely internally and externally

*Santosha* – contentment, gratitude

*Tapas* – austerity

*Swadhyaya* – study of religious text

*Iswara/pranindhana* – study of the sacred scriptures and elimination of ego.

When following the practice of the yamas and niyamas one will feel uplifted and elevated. This will help the yogi to prepare for a deeper, more purified meditation practice.

## Asanas

The word asana means postures or pose. Each and every posture in yoga has a Sanskrit name. Although the asanas are all hatha yoga based poses, the true meaning behind the word asana is literally 'seat'. When broken down, ha means sun and tha means moon. For example, a typical asana would be a lotus position. The yogi would sit in this posture for a pranayama and meditation practice. By participating in a yoga practice before taking your seat, the body will feel lose and supple, preparing you to sit still comfortably.

## Pranayama

The word pranayama has two parts: prana and ayama. Prana means vital life-force energy as in breath, life, energy and vitality. Ayama means expansion, lengthening, stretching or restraint. The two together means steady control of the breath.

These yogic breathing techniques are utilised during your yoga practice when you breathe rhythmically with each asana (posture), which will help purify and cleanse the body. It is also practiced before meditation to focus and calm the mind. Pranayama introduces the practitioner to pratyahara.

## Pratyahara

Pratyahara means 'to learn to withdraw from the senses by going deeply inward'. The practice of pratyahara leads to detachment from external objects. This means to no longer be fed by stimuli of our senses and be free from all their sensations. Being in this state of non-attachment results in restraints. Practicing this restraint neutralises habits and one's need to become dissipated.

This process usually happens when we are fully engrossed in our pranayama practice because the mind is so occupied with the breath. This state can be similar to the time we are about to fall asleep or upon awakening. It is when we have full awareness of what is going on; however, we are not distracted or influenced by it.

## Dharana

Dharana is the practice of mind concentration and learning to maintain proper concentration.

This can be achieved by fixating on an external object or an internal idea. This is a primary step in the process of mind control and preparation for higher meditational techniques.

## Dhyana

Dhyana can be defined as meditation. This is when one can devote oneself to an unbroken flow of awareness as a pure mental process. This continuous stream of one idea is not disturbed by any other thought.

## Samadhi

This is the super-conscious state of thinking and being, which is actually our natural spiritual state. In this intense state of 'being' or merging of the mind we can become at one with the whole oneness. When we succeed in samadhi, we are absorbed in something that becomes our stable unchanging reality. Samadhi is the goal that we are ultimately moving towards. Samadhi transcends time, space and causation.

Whereas the first five limbs explained above are a form of external yogic practice, the last three limbs represent entering a new internal yogic realm. When you constitute the last three, dharana, dhyana and samadhi these mean one has evolved to gain 'mastery' or 'unity'.

## Bhakti yoga

Bhakti is the devotional branch of yoga. Bhakti yoga can be practiced through prayer, chanting or the repetition of holy sacred syllables (japa). The daily practice of bhakti will bring about elimination of emotions connected to ego by helping to bring the focus to the heart centre through the practice of self-surrender and a loving attachment to the divine. The Sanskrit word bhakti derives from the root bhaj, which means to share, participate or worship. Bhajan is the name given to devotional singing or poetry. The Bhagavadgita (a sacred Hindu scripture) was one of the first texts to use the word bhakti.

## Karma yoga

Karma yoga means 'action' and it is the practice and dedication of selflessness without any thought of personal reward or expectation. Karma yoga is about offering yourself up and helping others by putting their needs first whether through acts of charity or helping to create a sense of community. Karma yoga can be practiced anywhere at any time regardless of conditions or circumstances. When the yogi participates in regular karma yoga, personal desires are banished and the heart is expanded. It is about living with humility and serving humanity, as well as other living beings such as animals and the planet.

Karma yoga can be practiced mentally as well as with the intention of taking action. Living your life by the karma yoga theory can feel very satisfying and liberating and free from fear. The yogi will have a big heart and be sincere in their help to others without any motive or discrimination. By donating selfless service you will purify your heart and gain an understanding of compassion, tolerance and empathy towards others. When one has developed pure love for others they will identify with the higher supreme self and annihilate selfishness and separation of the self. It truly represents the essence of opening up our hearts and seeing ourselves in others. Karma yoga is well complemented by bhakti yoga as one has to be devotional through the actions of karma.

*Bhakti* = emotional temperament

*Karma* = active temperament

## Jnana yoga

Jnana yoga, which is known as 'knowledge', is classified as the intellectual approach and the most direct of the four paths. Jnana teaches the yogi spiritual evolution or the 'absolute truth'. The yogi learns that liberation is attained not by works but only through knowledge. In order to learn jnana one has to be firmly grounded in the other three branches. The practice of jnana complements and balances with bhakti.

In jnana the yogi understands that our true self is behind and beyond our mind. This is self-realisation.

# Health benefits of yoga

Here is a list of some of the physiological and psychological benefits of yoga:

- Body becomes strong and supple

- Posture improves

- Balance improves

- Flexibility and agility increases

- Weight stabilises

- Restores youth

- Eye-hand coordination improves

- Balances the opposing muscle groups

- Immunity increases

- Respiratory efficiency increases

- Promotes deep sleep

- The mind is calmer and more relaxed

- Function of the endocrine system stabilises

- Promotes overall sense of feeling balanced and centred

- Reduces fatigue and weakness

- Anxiety and depression decrease

- Promotes well-being and vitality

- Attention and concentration improve

- Overall mood improves

- Boosts self-confidence

- Unlimited personal growth and self-awareness

- Better stress management

- Activates the parasympathetic nervous system (lowering blood pressure, slowing the pace of breathing and enables the body to relax and heal)

As this list is endless, I could go on. In fact, a whole book could be dedicated alone to the health benefits of practicing yoga.

# Breathing

I was at a Sivananda yoga teacher training course several years ago where I learnt that 80 per cent of your energy comes from breathing and only 20 per cent from food. We can live life without food and water for days however, if we are deprived of breathing, our life would end in minutes. It is imperative to breathe correctly so the human body can function properly. Correct breathing makes sure all the organs and cells are enriched with a fresh supply of oxygen.

When we lead hectic lifestyles in today's modern society, our breathing patterns become a true reflection of how we conduct our life.

Have you noticed when you are rushing around like a maniac or worried about something that your breathing pattern changes to 'shallow breath' or you're not even able to catch the breath at all due to anxiety? It is these moments that we need to really pay attention to the breath and have more of a conscious control over it.

To breathe correctly, one needs to inhale expanding the diaphragm. This is where the inhalation starts which leads up to the intercostal muscles and finally the clavicle area. Unfortunately, most people only breathe shallowly, through the clavicle area, thus lifting the shoulders and not activating the lower part of the body. If your breathing pattern becomes shallow, the rest of the body does not get enough fresh oxygen to reach all the cells, resulting in a poor immune system and lack of vitality. Breathing shallowly can also irritate the top of the lungs and constrict your full capacity to breathe correctly.

This is why in yoga the breath is stipulated as a very dominant part of the yogic practice. Many breathing techniques have been devised to teach the practitioner to learn to control 'prana' (vital life force energy), which leads to learning to control the mind.

*When the breath wanders, the mind is unsteady, but when the breath is still, so is the mind still.*

Hatha yoga pradipika

# Pranayama terms and breathing techniques

## Ujjayi

This breathing technique can be practised in a seated, upright, cross-legged position or it can be applied with the yoga postures. I always tell my students to take a deep inhalation and exhalation through the nostrils. It is on the exhalation that you contract the upper throat in the glottis to create an 'h' sound like at the seashore or even like Darth Vader. The exhalation should feel natural without force or nasally.

### Benefits

Ujjayi is known to raise the body heat, which helps purify and dissolve toxins. It performs internal purification, activation and energises conditioning all at the same time. One of the most beneficial properties of this technique is that many asthmatics have reaped great rewards and healed from ujjayi as it strengthens the condition of the lungs and the bronchiole linings. It also stimulates the 'digestive fire'.

## Kapalabhati

This means 'shining skull' and is considered a cleansing technique for the whole of the respiratory system. It is one of the six 'kriyas' (in Sanskrit this means action, deed, effort), which is known as a cleansing practice in hatha yoga.

You can perform this in a seated position. It is ideal first thing in the morning preferably outside.

The exhalation is short, sharp and very forceful through the nose. As you pump the stomach muscles in and out, imagine you are blowing out a candle or blowing your nose through the nostrils. The inhalation is very passive, however you must remember to catch the inhalation otherwise you run out of breath. Start with about three rounds of 20–30 pumps and gradually build up to five rounds of 100 pumps.

### Benefits

This style of breathing is very energising and great if you're feeling tired and need a natural tonic. This will help boost the oxygen supply and purify the blood. It helps get rid of any stagnant air from the bottom of the lungs due to incorrect, shallow, breathing. It also helps to tone up the stomach muscles and leaves you feeling radiant and revitalised.

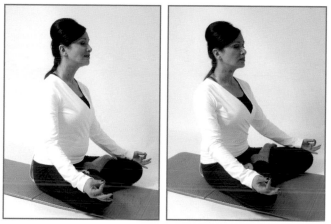

*Kapalabhati*

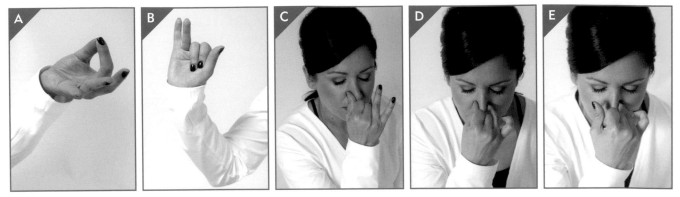

*Anuloma viloma*

## Anuloma viloma

Anuloma viloma or alternate nostril breathing is a technique where you inhale through one nostril and exhale out of the other. The practitioner usually applies this method before a meditation practice to focus the mind on one-pointedness (complete concentration on one object). Sitting down cross-legged, take your left hand to 'chi mudra' (picture A) and take your right hand to 'vishnu mudra' (picture B).

Rest your left hand on top of the left knee. On the right hand, fold down the index and middle fingers. Close the right nostril with your thumb (picture C) and exhale completely through the left nostril. Inhale completely through the left nostril keeping the right side closed and now also close off the left nostril and retain the breath (picture D).

The inhalation should last four counts, retain for 16 counts and exhale for eight counts. Repeat this to the other side, this time exhale out of the right nostril, keeping the left side blocked off (picture E). Inhale through the right and retain the breath again. Keep repeating this beginning with five rounds (each side is one round) and build up to ten. This technique is best practised after kapalabhati (see previous page).

### Benefits

Alternate nostril breathing helps to balance the two hemispheres of the brain (male and female energy). It is

medically known that at any one time our nasal cycle will favour one side and be more prominent from breathing in and out of that same side for up to three hours. The yoga science had discovered this thousands of years ago and therefore devised this particular breathing technique to help re-establish the natural nasal cycle, which clears the blockage by regulating the airflow. Disturbances of the nasal cycle over a long period of time signals poor balance and functioning of the breath, leading to disease. In this technique, the retention of the breath will increase more pressure, so the exchange of gaseous air becomes greater, therefore one not only gets rid of $CO_2$ on the exhalation but other toxins held in the body will also be eliminated.

These breathing techniques (and Anuloma viloma in particular) are all believed to purify and cleanse the nadis. The nadis are equivalent to what is known in western terms as the meridians or energy channels in our body. We have 72,000 nadis in our subtle body. However, the three main ones which stand out are the ida, the pingala with the main one being the sushumna.

The sushumna channel runs through the spinal cord starting at the base of the spine all the way to the crown of the head. The pingala nadi is on the right side of the body. It is the male energy, which is connected to the solar/sun (heat). The ida nadi is on the left-hand side of the body and is connected to the lunar/moon (cool). When these two energy channels are in union with one another, they send a flow of prana flowing upwards through the sushumna canal. This energetic current is known to activate the kundalini energy. This is a coiled serpent-like energy that lies dormant in the base of the spine.

* *Stop all these techniques if you start to feel light-headed or dizzy.*
* *Please remember that these breathing techniques are not suitable if you're pregnant.*

# The three bandhas

The word bandha means lock. Locks are used in various asanas and pranayama practices to energise and cleanse the internal organs of the body.

When assimilated, bandhas interconnect the inner systems in the internal subtle energy and bind the energy from leaking out to move it upwards to restrain the downward order of energy.

It is important to know these bandhas are not viewed as muscle contractions. When these bandha techniques are practiced, it awakens the psychic energy known as kundalini. When this kundalini energy is activated through the practice of pranayama and the application of the bandhas, this natural conscious energy of the self brings the practitioner to an enlightened state of being.

## Mula bandha

Mula bandha is the root energy which flows between the body and the earth. When applying this bandha during a practice of yoga and meditation, the aim is to contract the anal sphincter and squeeze the pelvic floor by drawing the energy upwards towards the abdominals which naturally leads to the next lock uddiyana bandha. This movement by no means represents a pelvic tilt (anterior or posterior rotation of the pelvis). This action occurs deep within the energetic moveable elements of the pelvic girdle.

## Uddiyana bandha

Uddiyana bandha means the energy flying upwards. Practiced alone or in conjunction with the mula bandha it massages and cleanses the abdominal organs. This lock is used to control the flow of breath and energy in the body while in a yoga practice. It will help increase the power of the core enabling the practitioner to hold a steady balance of the postures more successfully.

As a pranayama practice, this lock can be very strenuous yet energising. To practice this, one has to empty the lungs with a forceful exhalation. This will make the diaphragm rise naturally in the thoracic region. Finally, you draw the intestines and the navel area towards the back so the abdominals rest against the thoracic cavity.

## Jalandhara bandha

Jalandhara is known as the chin lock. In some postures in yoga this happens naturally due to the positioning of the posture as in, for example, sarvangasasna (shoulder stand). In pranayama, this lock is usually applied on the retention of the breath by placing the tongue against the roof of the mouth to create a vacuum at the back of the throat. At the same time press your chin in towards the chest.

When performing these three bandhas for pranayama techniques the practitioner can be in a seated cross-legged position (padmasana or sukasana). Alternatively, depending on which 'kriya' you are practicing, you may stand up. When all these three locks are held in the body at the same time this is known as 'maha bandhu'. If you are a beginner trying these, start only holding the retention for a few seconds at a time. These are not recommended if you are pregnant.

# The chakras

The word chakra derives from the Sanskrit word 'cakra' or spinning wheel or circle. Chakras come from the ancient tantric yoga tradition. These are known as the subtle energy centres. These spinning vortices of light, colour and frequency are openings for energy to flow in and out of the aura.

Chakras are a good indicator of how the body functions on an energetic level. If all the seven chakras are not in harmony with one another, the others have to work harder to compensate and to create balance.

Each chakra corresponds to a different area of the body. The usual locations are in a straight line from the base of the spine (root chakra) to the top of the head (crown chakra). The lower three chakras correspond to the physical body, while the top three relate to our intuition, communication, creativity and consciousness. The heart chakra in the centre bridges the top and bottom chakras.

## The seven chakras

▸ **Sahasrara** – crown chakra

▸ **Ajna** – third eye chakra

▸ **Vishuddha** – throat chakra – ether element

▸ **Anahata** – heart centre chakra – air element

▸ **Manipura** – solar plexus chakra – fire element

▸ **Swadhisthana** – sacral chakra – water element

▸ **Muladhara** – root chakra – earth element

The crown chakra, sahasrara, represents the ultimate connection of your physical body to the spiritual realm. It is about achieving oneness with the universe and the highest state of divinity. The headstand is a good posture for this chakra.

The third eye chakra, ajna, is connected with the colour indigo. This is an etheric organ which is located between the eyebrows. When awake this chakra is recognised as the doorway to wisdom and supreme consciousness. It is known to activate creativity as well as seeing physically a broader perspective of life. It is a way of living your life intuitively. This chakra is great for penetrating insight and knowledge. Meditation and alternate nostril breathing is good for the activation of this chakra.

The throat chakra, vishuddha, is blue and associated with communication. This represents honesty of expression and openness. It is about being truthful and sincere with your words.

The heart chakra, anahata, is seen as green. This chakra emanates love. The feelings associated with this chakra are from virtuous emotions such as compassion, joy, happiness, understanding, generosity and selflessness. The fish pose is great for this chakra.

The solar plexus, manipura chakra, is yellow. This part of the body is a direct link to a person's emotional life. This is the life force or seat of your body's battery. If this part of your body is blocked, one cannot connect to oneself on a deeper level and lacks purpose. The best pose for this is the bow.

The sacral chakra, swadhisthana, is associated with the colour orange. It is situated just below the navel and it has to do with learning to lessen control issues and knowing how to 'let go'. It is mainly associated with the reproductive organs and corresponds with bodily functions such as sexuality and reproduction.

The root chakra, muladhara, is connected to the colour red. This root chakra is the grounding force which is the base for all the other chakras and our connection to the earth. It is located in the perineum where the kundalini energy sits. It is about you as it defines your core self and your life as in your survival. This is why it is recommended to sit down in meditation so that one can make that instant connection to the earth's energy.

# Yoga demonstration

Here I demonstrate a variety of yoga postures which I use regularly in my own personal yoga practice and also teach in my classes. As I have been trained in two disciplines, hatha (Sivananda style) and Ashtanga (primary series, Mysore style) some of the postures will derive from these two styles of yoga.

The sequence of these postures is not necessarily in any particular order, however, I have, where possible, tried to use counter postures so that you work opposite muscle groups as in lengthening and contraction. When teaching these postures in the correct sequence from their original method of practice, each pose will usually start from one posture and sometimes flow into another depending on the style of yoga.

Please note: this is just a brief explanation and summary of the postures and not a full comprehensive and detailed guide.

Each posture has a series of steps that help you to manoeuvre into the end pose. All the postures would usually have variations for all levels of practitioners. As a general guideline though, if you are a beginner and are trying the postures for the first few times, please go into them gently and slowly. Try not to force your body into any of the positions as you will create more tension. The whole aim is to think about surrendering the body and letting it get into the positions more naturally. I recommend after finishing the surya-namuskar (sun salutations), which will warm up the body, you begin the asanas (postures). If you are a beginner, you hold each pose for five deep breaths. More advanced practitioners may hold the pose for one minute or longer for a stronger practice.

Women who are menstruating should avoid the inverted poses (legs up in the air) as you are affecting the natural flow of prana (vital life force energy). All the asanas will help tone and strengthen all the muscles and make the joints more supple and the whole body loose and flexible.

The practice of all these postures will not only help the physical body but through using the breath rhythmically with each posture, your mind will calm down and stay more focused, especially on the balancing postures where one needs to remain present.

It is well documented from the yoga gurus that the three main asanas that are a must in any yoga practice is the headstand, the shoulder stand and the seated forward bend. However, completing the whole practice will aid mental awareness and spiritual well-being.

> **Note:** you will notice that nearly all yogic postures end in asana.

# Surya-namaskar

## Sun salutation

Surya-namaskar, or sun salutations, are a series of 12 postures performed in a graceful flow. Each movement is coordinated with the breath. There are many varied styles of sun salutations depending on which discipline one is practicing. These 12 steps always start at the beginning of a yoga practice to warm up and stimulate the muscles and the spinal column. Usually each pose will counteract the other with a vertebral movement to promote flexibility.

The great thing about this sequence is that it caters for all levels and everyone can try them, including the elderly and children, as it is a natural way to warm up the body physically and physiologically. There are modifications if you are pregnant.

Start by standing with your feet together and ground the heels, staying centred. Tuck your tailbone under, close your eyes for a few seconds and connect to the breath. Once you have created a calm space, remain present and make the breath the intention. Start by having the hands in namaste (prayer position), in front of the heart centre.

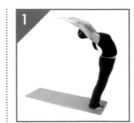

▶ Inhale, stretch up, arch back. Make sure you keep the head in line with your arms. Your arms should be alongside the ears and fingers closed to keep the energy in the body.

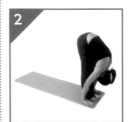

▶ Exhale, folding forwards. As you fold forwards place the palms of your hands around the outside of your feet so that hands and feet are all aligned with one another. If you find it difficult to reach the floor, then bend the knees.

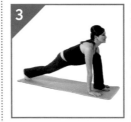

▶ Inhale, lunge back with the right leg keeping the hands firmly in the same place throughout the rest of the sequence. Make sure your back is not rounded, squeeze the shoulder blades together and open up the chest by looking upwards. Make sure that you are not putting too much tension on the knee on the front leg and that it is not going over the toes.

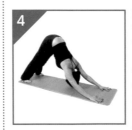

▶ Exhale into a downward facing dog. When performing this stance, make sure you iron out the crease in the thoracic (upper) region of the spine by drawing the chest towards the knees as you exhale. Make sure your fingertips are spread evenly so that the skin of the thumb and index finger is firmly pressed down with the same pressure as the other three fingers. Gaze into the solar plexus (stomach) and lift your tailbone as high as you can.

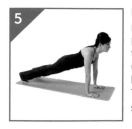

▶ Inhale to the plank (push up) position. When you are holding this pose, push your body weight down into the heels and apply the lower bandhas (see page 45). Make sure your lower back does not sink towards the floor. The body should remain in a long straight line.

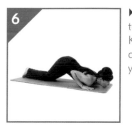

▶ Exhale, knees, chest, forehead down to the floor keeping the gaze ahead. Keep the hips lifted off the floor. If you are a beginner at this, you may rest your forehead on the floor.

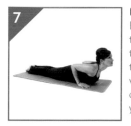

▶ Inhale, slide forward into bhujanganasana (cobra). As you slide the body forwards until the hips touch the ground, gaze upwards and keep the hands in the same position the whole time. Arch the back and push down the shoulder blades by taking your shoulders away from the ears.

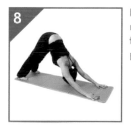

▶ Exhale, tuck the toes under without moving the hands into a downward facing dog. Use the same teaching points as before (see image 4).

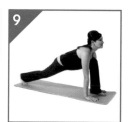

▶ Inhale, lunge forward with your left leg. Use the same teaching points as position 3.

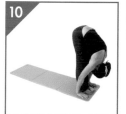

▶ Exhale, without moving the hands bring both legs together, drawing nose to knee (same as position 2).

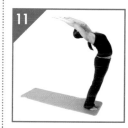

▶ Inhale stretch up and arch back, as you stretch upwards here, imagine someone is standing in front of you, holding your hands and pulling you forward so that your arms are making a scooping action upwards.

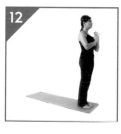

▶ Exhale, bring your arms to the heart centre in the prayer position and get ready to go again.

This time you will lead with the left leg and come back on the right leg. One round of sun salutations means performing once on each leg. Please start with five rounds and eventually build up to 12 rounds.

# THE ASANAS

## Pada hastasana

Hands to feet pose

### benefits ›

Pada hastasana, or hands to feet pose, is highly beneficial for lengthening the entire back of the body. This aids in promoting flexibility for the spine and especially the hamstrings. As the head is below the heart, there is an increased flow of blood to the brain.

### tips ›

Keep the heels fully grounded and make sure your body weight is in the balls of the feet and the legs remain active.

# Trikonasana

## The triangle

### benefits ›

Trikonasana, or the triangle, is a very well-known and practised posture within a hatha or Ashtanga yoga based class. It will help to promote hip and leg flexibility. The posture gives a stretch to both sides of the body and a lateral stretch to both sides of the spine too. This will help the spine to remain elastic.

The chest is also relaxed and expanded in this posture. Altogether this pose creates a good steady balance.

### tips ›

Make sure both legs are fully extended so the flesh above the knee is lifted and the upper thigh muscles contracted as you hold this posture. The shoulders should stack on top of each other and the arms straight going away from each other as though someone is pulling your arms in a long straight line. Bring your gaze up to your fingers.

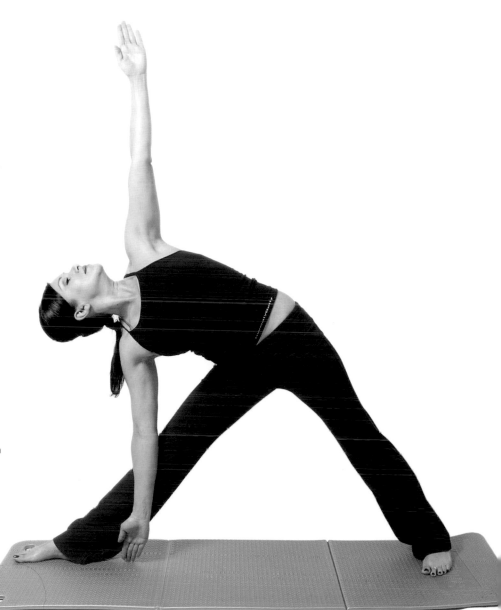

# Prasarita padottanasana

## Wide-legged forward bend

### benefits ›

Prasarita padottanasana, or wide-legged forward bend, strengthens and stretches the inner thighs, hamstrings and the spine. This posture also helps to tone the stomach muscles and relieves back tension.

In some yoga disciplines it is used as a preparation for a tripod headstand variation.

### tips ›

**The finger grip**

Slide the index and middle fingers between the big toes and the second toes so the fingertips are going inwards. Curl your fingers under and grab the big toes firmly, wrapping your thumbs around the two fingers to secure a grip. If you have an existing lower back problem, avoid the full bend until your back is stronger.

If your head does not touch the ground use a block and place the crown of the head on the block

or alternatively, if you can't reach your toes, use a strap by placing it under the balls of each feet and pull the straps towards you as you lean forward.

Keep the weight centred in the balls of the feet and spine as long as possible.

Keep the lower bandhas in the body engaged, paying special attention to uddiyana bandha (stomach lock) to keep your balance.

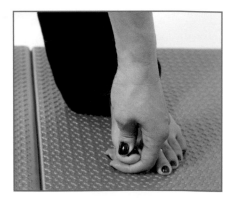

# Parivrtta parsvakonasana

## Revolving side angle

### benefits ›

Parivrtta parsvakonasana, or revolving side angle, is probably one of the most challenging yet powerful asanas.

As this pose involves a twist, you are deeply working on the internal organs. This posture is very effective for getting rid of blockages and helps shift energy in the solar plexus area (stomach). As the solar plexus is connected to all your feelings and emotions such as fear, anxiety, anger etc, the revolving twist helps to get the digestive fire going through the breath (ujjayi). This will generate heat in the body helping digestion and remove the blockage whether physical or emotional. This posture really makes the practitioner stay present in order to maintain a steady balance. The posture helps to strengthen the shoulders, spine and all surrounding muscles. Also this will open up the chest, groin and hip flexors.

### tips ›

If you are new to this posture, instead of a bind with the arms, take your hands in prayer position and drop your back leg down so your knee is touching the floor. If however, your back leg is off the floor, you may push your weight right back into your heel to establish a good firm base.

# Virabhadrasana

## The warrior

### benefits ›

Virabhadrasana, or the warrior, is very well-known as the name for a fierce warrior. This powerful asana strengthens the legs, ankles and hip flexors. It also stretches the inner thigh, groin, chest, shoulders and helps correct painful conditions around the sacrum. You will notice an improvement in your concentration from regular practise of this posture.

### tips ›

Keep your feet firmly grounded, lifting everything from the hip upwards. Keep the lower bandhas engaged (mula and uddiyana bandhas). Look forward, bringing your gaze over the top of the fingertips.

# Vrikshasana

## The tree

### benefits ›

Vrikshasana, or the tree, is a balancing posture which helps cultivate a better sense of feeling centred. It helps improve respiration and strengthens the thighs, ankles, calves and spine.

### tips ›

When you're trying to keep your balance in this posture, find a fixed spot on the floor and concentrate all your efforts on staying focused on this point. As well as keeping focus, you can visualise yourself in the posture in your mind's eye as you're in the stance. Also, you can establish a solid base by rooting your leg down and connecting it to the earth just like a tree. This goes back to manifesting your thoughts through visualisation. Keep the breath steady and relaxed. Beginners initially may use something to hold onto for support.

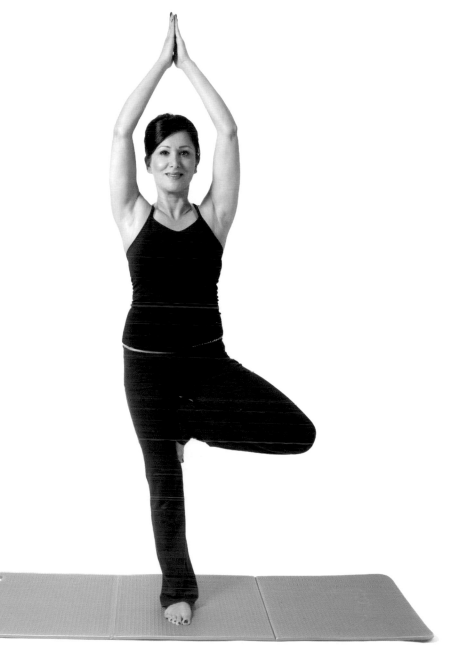

# Kakasana

## The crow

### benefits ›

The kakasana, or the crow, is another challenging balancing posture which really demands a still mind and concentration through steady breath. It helps strengthen the wrists, arms and shoulders.

It helps promote physical and mental balance and a sense of calmness.

### tips ›

The most important tip for this asana is to keep your gaze ahead to avoid rolling forwards and gently allow yourself to get into the full posture.

# Dhanurasana

## The bow

### benefits ›

Dhanurasana, or the bow, is a very beneficial asana for the entire spine. It helps improve all areas of the spine – lumber, thoracic and cervical (lower, upper and back of neck area). This posture will also help stimulate the digestive organs by giving an invigorated massage to all the organs. Your back will feel open and energised after this asana.

### tips ›

When going into this posture, it is important to remember to lift your ankles up with your arms. Most people lift up their chest first and the aim is to use the strength of your upper body to get the height in the legs. Legs should be apart. Beginners should try one leg up on one side at a time if you cannot clasp your ankles.

# Pachimothasana

## Seated-forward bend

### benefits ▸

Pachimothasana, or seated-forward bend, is an asana which is recognised and almost always used in any yoga discipline. If you have a limited yoga practice, then this posture is a must. It is the posture of surrender. If all the asanas had to be a type of food, then this posture would be a superfood. This asana helps to lengthen the hamstrings and stretch the lumbar region of the spine giving a massage to the stomach. The spine remains elastic and joints become mobile from regular practice of this posture.

### tips ▸

When you come forwards into the bend, try and lead from the base of the spine keeping the chest open, avoiding restriction, otherwise you will get a rounded back. Push your weight back into your tailbone as you reach forward and relax into the posture effortlessly.

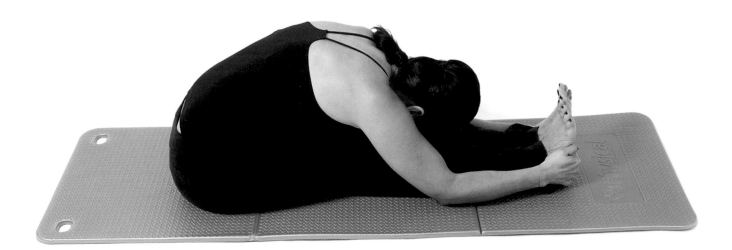

# Chakrasana

## The wheel pose

### benefits ›

Chakrasana, or the wheel pose, is a strong posture that improves the suppleness, strength and the elasticity of the spinal cord. This pose opens up the chest and promotes deep steady breathing to help expand the lungs.

In general this posture has an overall tonic effect on the whole body and boosts energy, which stimulates all the functioning systems of the body.

### tips ›

This posture is very much aimed at the advanced practitioner, therefore if your back needs to get more flexible before you attempt this, you can try a bridge pose. This involves lifting the lower part of your body (hips and pelvis), keeping the head and shoulders on the ground. Interlace your arms on the floor behind your back to start with.

# Sirsasana

## The headstand

### benefits ▸

Sirsasana, also known as the headstand, is another powerful inversion. Sometimes known as the king of all asanas. As you are upside down in this posture, it enhances deep breathing, bringing an increased supply of oxygen to the brain. The headstand has many physiological and physical benefits. While upside down this helps your mind to calm down through the concentration of the posture. This also helps improve mental power and increase your self-confidence. I always think when you go upside down that all your insecurities fall out of your pockets. It's also a great way to boost the strength in your arms and shoulders.

### tips ▸

In this posture, make sure that most of your weight (90 per cent) is in your arms and not pressing on the head. Please make sure that your elbows are narrower than your shoulders. Beginners should practise by taking only one leg up and down at a time or use a wall as support. Avoid this if you suffer from high blood pressure. Always rest in the child's pose after the headstand.

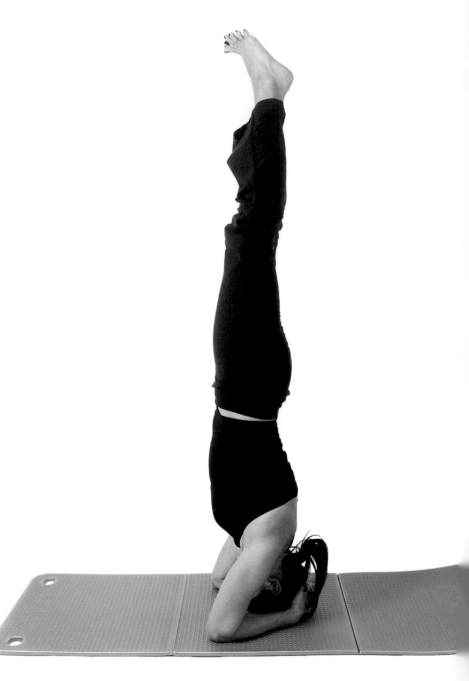

# Balasana

## The child's pose

### benefits ›

Balasana, or the child's pose, derives its name from the word bala which means child in Sanskrit. This is a restorative posture which helps calm the mind and gather the breath. A gentle stretch is given to the thighs and hips. The muscle tendons and ligaments in the knee are also stretched. As your head is lower than your heart, you receive more circulation to your face. It is a very relaxing and therapeutic posture which helps relieve tension, anxiety and stress.

### tips ›

This is the posture where you can really let go and surrender the body to deeply feel relaxed.

During a yoga practice, if you need to rest at any time due to fatigue, a child's pose is highly recommended.

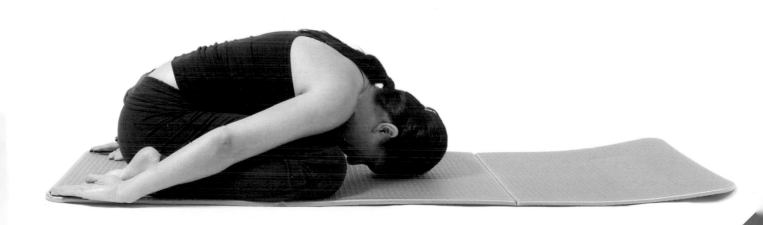

# Sarvangasana

## The shoulder stand

### benefits ›

Sarvangasana, or the shoulder stand, has many benefits, the main one being that this posture helps regulate and stimulate the thyroid gland whether it's over- or under-active. The thyroid is the most important gland in our endocrine system (which produces hormones). It helps balance the body's metabolic rate and heat production. Weight issues deriving from a poorly functioning thyroid will be a cause of imbalance.

The third bandha (jalandhara) is engaged in the posture encouraging the practitioner to breathe correctly starting at the diaphragm. This posture is excellent for relieving fatigue and makes you mentally alert.

### tips ›

If your back does not feel flexible enough to extend your legs all the way up or your upper body does not have the strength to support you, then use a wall to walk your legs up. If you have neck problems avoid this asana all together.

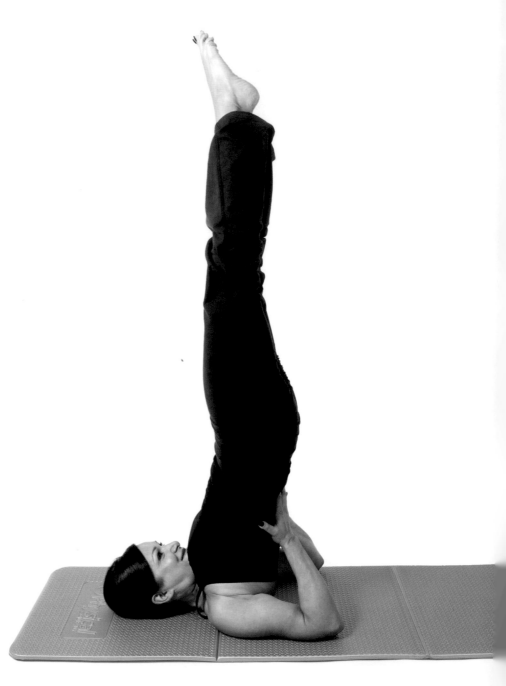

# Matsyasana

## The fish pose

### benefits ▸

Matsyasana, or the fish, is known in yogic text as the posture that is the 'destroyer of all diseases'.

It is a great posture for really opening up and expanding the heart centre. It helps stimulate and stretch the belly, throat and neck and strengthen the upper back and the back of the neck.

### tips ▸

By holding this pose and bringing your awareness to the heart centre through the breath, one can help shift and remove physical and emotional blockages. Avoid this if you have a neck injury.

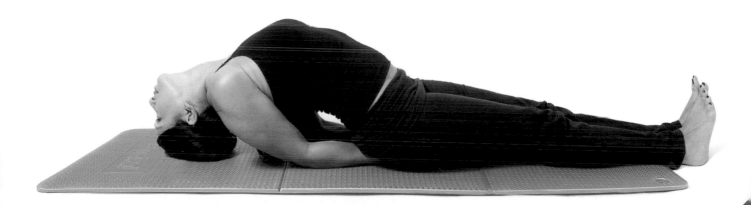

# Savasana

## The corpse pose

### benefits ›

Savasana, or the corpse pose, is recognised as the final relaxation in any yoga practice and may last from 5–15 minutes (the longer the better). It helps rejuvenate and refresh the body after a lengthy or deep practice. It is the perfect cool down that helps the body to settle and relax. Proper relaxation is essential for the health of the body and mind.

### tips ›

During this section of the class make sure you wrap up warm because your body temperature starts to drop as you cool down. Really let the body and mind go completely to have a peaceful rest. However, it is important to stay conscious to reap the full benefits as it is very easy to fall asleep.

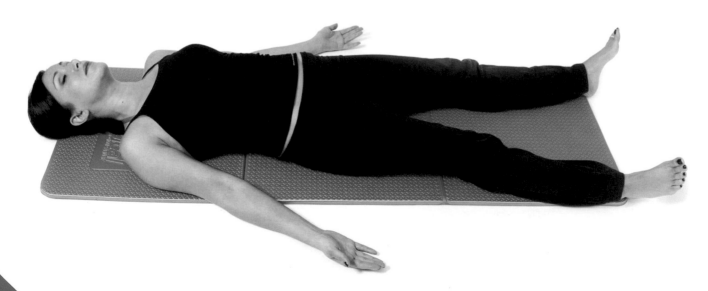

# Padmasana

## The lotus pose

### benefits ›

Padmasana, or lotus, is probably one of the most recognised postures generally. It is the main seated posture for meditation or pranayama practice. This posture is ancient and because of the lengthy time spent sitting in this pose, the sages created yoga so that their bodies became loose and supple enough for them to do this without any discomfort. Make sure you keep the spine long and neck tall during your practice. It is a great position for maintaining full awareness of an upright posture. Support the back by locking the lower bundhas.

### tips ›

This is an advanced posture, therefore an alternative option would be to try sukasana, which is sitting upright in a cross-legged position. Some people may even find that difficult so you can sit upright in a chair for a meditation practice, however, the seated posture is recommended. When first sitting down in this posture, use a cushion for support for your back. Make sure your sitting bones are grounded into the cushion and feel a real sense of connection to the earth. Plug into the earth's energy and visualise it coming up the spine, through to the neck and up to the crown of the head.

# Styles of yoga classes

## Hatha yoga

This is slow-paced and more of a gentle practice, making it great for newcomers to this style of yoga. The postures are usually held longer. The class will usually be taught simple breathing methods and meditation.

## Ashtanga yoga

This kind of class was created by Sri Pattabhi Jois and the poses are usually performed in a 'vinyasa flow style' (breath synchronised movement). This practice usually involves using ujjayi, breathing techniques and the bandhas. Ashtanga is more physically demanding because it is based on the flow of moving from one pose to another without pause.

## Iyengar yoga

This yoga practice was created by B K S Iyengar and is a form of hatha-based poses while paying special attention to posture alignment. It normally involves using props such as straps, blocks, blankets and bolsters. In Iyengar you will hold the poses for longer periods.

## Bikram yoga

Bikram yoga or 'hot yoga' is recognised for practicing in a room where the temperature is 105°F (40°C) with 40 per cent humidity. It is a 90-minute practice with a sequence of 26 hatha-based postures and two breathing techniques.

## Power yoga

This class is really popular with the Westerners who prefer an athletic and vigorous work-out. It is much more fitness orientated. It uses the postures of the Ashtanga style of yoga, however, not necessarily in a particular sequence.

## Jivamukti yoga

This style of yoga, which is one I personally practice, is a more modern style of yoga using Ashtanga and Vinyasa-style practices. Even though it is physically challenging, it is balanced with the traditional yoga features such as chanting, yoga scripture, meditating and pranayama.

# Meditation

## What is meditation?

Meditation can have many different definitions. However, a conventional meditation practice usually means sitting in silence and calming the mind.

Many students come to my classes and tell me that they find it impossible to clear their mind, as their head is too consumed with thoughts and noise. It is these people who actually need it the most.

As for the part about completely clearing the mind, well it is almost impossible to just sit down, close your eyes and stop the thoughts; and that is not the point anyway.

The whole point of meditation is initially to sit in silence. Gently close your eyes and connect to the breath. Start to witness and observe your thoughts just as though you're watching a movie. This in itself is a form of meditation and a starting point to having awareness of what thoughts you are having. When your thoughts come up, try not to get attached or engaged with them. Simply acknowledge them and let them go. This will help the mind to focus and concentrate on being in the present moment. This is the first part to clearing the mind.

The second part is to breathe deeply so that every cell in your body will get a fresh supply of oxygenated rich air; hence the calming effect on the mind. The deep breathing will cleanse the respiratory system and calm the nervous system.

Once the body and mind start to calm down, you will eventually find you will have gaps and spaces between your thinking. This is a sign that the body has gone into deeper relaxation. If you associate a certain smell with this state, such as incense or burning a candle/oil, then you will find that your body will naturally adapt to this mind state a lot quicker. This is also achieved by having a routine of when you do your practice, such as first thing in the morning, and by sitting in the same place. As your body familiarises itself with this routine, this will help you get into that serene peaceful state quicker.

Another way to become calm is to have a mantra, for example, breathing in 'let' and breathing out 'go' so that you can bring the focus into something more internal and help to withdraw your senses deeply within and connect to the self. Usually, I encourage my class to bring their internal gaze up to the point between their eyebrows known as the 'third eye' centre (ajna chakra). This will activate the pineal gland, which is the doorway to cosmic consciousness and creativity. In yoga this chakra is known to be connected to mysticism and psychic awareness.

Like anything else, the more you practise, the better your meditation practice will become. Remember, when you first sit and close your eyes dedicate yourself to being still and allow whatever needs to, to come up. Sometimes you will be surprised at what you are witnessing but these are things that have manifested themselves and have clearly come up for a reason.

## What are the benefits?

The health benefits of meditation are endless as it is an overall tonic for every aspect of your health, which in turn helps every facet of your life. It really is a process of self-discovery to get to know the 'real you' because it teaches you to connect to the true essence of yourself. Once you know yourself, you know others. When you peel off the layers of perceived identity, as in sibling, partner, parent, profession etc, true realisation and purpose reveals itself.

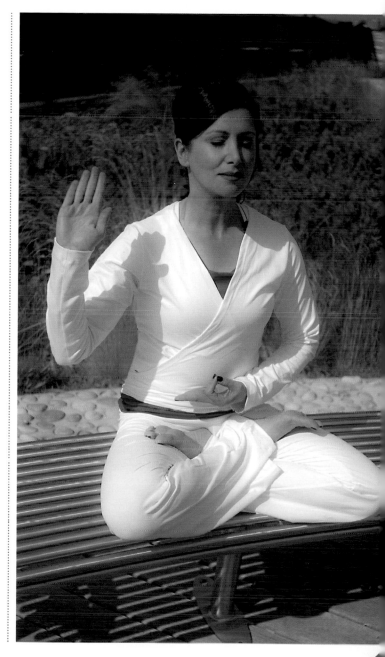

Here are some of the benefits of meditation:

▶ The cells in the body receive more oxygen and other nutrients are absorbed in abundance.

▶ It improves concentration as it strengthens the mind. For example, professional athletes have seen sports performance levels increase immensely due to a regular meditation practice.

▶ It is a great medicine for reducing stress as poor health is usually a result of the manifestation of inner turmoil.

▶ It increases the activity of 'natural killer cells' which destroy bacteria and cancerous cells. Remember, disease does not survive in oxygen.

▶ As it makes the immune system stronger and lowers blood lactate levels, this helps reduce anxiety.

▶ It increases the blood flow and slows down the heart rate, which helps regulate the blood pressure.

▶ It stimulates serotonin levels. Serotonin is known as the 'happy' hormone found naturally in the human brain. Serotonin is responsible for transmitting nerve impulses.

▶ In general, someone who practices meditation for a long period of time has a much calmer and relaxed outlook on life.

▶ If you are a sufferer of PMT (pre-menstrual tension), there has been a direct link showing that meditation helps reduce the erratic thought-patterns which accompany the symptoms. As you meditate, the mind quietens and you become less attached to irrational thoughts, thus balancing the emotions.

# Various styles of meditation

There are many different ways to meditate. Whichever style you adopt, I recommend you meditate twice a day for 20 minutes if you really want to reap the benefits.

In my own personal practice, I start first thing in the morning. I have been doing this for over seven years now and the results are indescribable. All I can say is that if I miss out on my practice, I don't feel centred or grounded. You could go as far as saying that my feet don't even connect with the earth as my head is spinning. The best word to describe a lack of practice for myself would be that I feel totally discombobulated.

I have integrated meditation, just as I have exercise, into my life as systematically as eating, sleeping and brushing my teeth. It is a daily activity which I cannot live without.

When I sit to meditate, I always burn an incense stick so my mind associates that smell with a relaxed state. I go into a trance state straight away from this. I start with two pranayama techniques, kapalabhati and alternate nostril breathing. As I have a more prominent connection to my male energy, I find the latter very balancing. After these

two techniques, which can take me up to ten minutes, my mind feels calm even though I feel very alert and awake. It is important to stay present and not run away with your thoughts or get connected to your feelings. Personally, I finish my last ten minutes of practice by doing some transcendental meditation. This means I repeat a mantra and focus my mind by listening to music with the sound of drums or I listen to nature sounds, such as birds.

Another form of meditation is to sit still and observe the breath only. Pay attention to how the breath enters the body on the inhalation and which nostril is it predominantly coming in through. Keep your awareness on the exhalation by feeling whether the breath is hot or cool.

Alternatively, you can sit down and make the intention of your meditation practice journeying. This means, through visualisation using the mind's eye. You can imagine, for instance, that you're on a beautiful, hot beach and you are listening to the healing sounds of the sea. You will feel the difference in your body, internally and externally. Or choose whichever location appeals to you.

There is one form of meditation which in yoga is called tratak. It is an excellent exercise to make your vision stronger too. You need to light a candle and sit down and watch the flame without closing your eyes for as long as you can. This really enhances your concentration. While you're watching the flame if a thought comes up, instantly let it go and start counting in your head, each time a thought comes up, start counting from one again until eventually, you can keep counting as your processed thoughts have slowed down and diminished.

# Mantra

A mantra can be a powerful word or affirmation which you repeat silently or loud, either during a meditation practice to distract the mind or in everyday life. It can be a sound like 'om' which is a holy sacred syllable commonly used in eastern theologies such as Hinduism or Buddhism.

# Meditation and brainwave frequencies

Our brainwaves use electricity called neurons to communicate with each other. The neurons are made of billions of cells which make up the brain to send out millions of signals at once. These signals create massive electrical currents in the brain, which can be measured using sensitive equipment called EEG (electroencephalogram). These emanating currents of electrical activity have different brainwave frequencies.

Through the practice of meditation, one can achieve a certain type of frequency which enables the practitioner to heal themselves and be open to creative consciousness. This is how one connects to the resource of higher infinite power. In the previous chapter of this book, we spoke about the subconscious. This is also a powerful state to be in in order to re-programme the sub-conscious by feeding it with sublime thoughts. Let me explain these frequencies.

## Beta

Beta frequency is when the brain is aroused and engaged in mental activity. It is when the focus and attention of the mind is directed more outward and consciously alert. Most people function in this frequency in their daily everyday tasks at work only when they are not in auto pilot mode.

## Gamma

There is a faster brainwave frequency than beta that is called gamma. This measures as the fastest brainwave and is associated with when a person is highly conscious and even more mentally active. It is also known that truly experienced meditators (monks) have this brainwave frequency mostly stimulated when the levels of consciousness are raised and the third eye centre (ajna chakra) is activated.

## Alpha

Alpha frequency is when your mind starts to relax by going more inward, yet you are still fully conscious and aware of what is happening around you. When one is reflecting, whether in nature or at the beginning of a meditation practice, brainwaves will be in this frequency.

## Theta

Theta frequency is associated with a dream or fantasy state. This can also be known as the hypnotic state. When the brainwaves are much slower and calmer your creativity kicks in and inspiring ideas start flowing in from a higher source. This is a very positive mental state to be in. Being in this frequency allows you to heal and change the subconscious mind. Through meditative development, one has the ability to remain conscious while going into this deeper state and changing the brainwave frequency to theta.

## Delta

Delta consciousness is the unconscious state. It is perhaps known as being at one with the whole and no longer identifying with the physical body. It is a state of non-duality. If you maintain your consciousness between theta and delta, you can transcend the laws of the physical world because you're not bound by them any more.

# Ayurvedic medicine

Ayurvedic is a scientific methodology using natural healing medicine. This ancient system derived from the Hindu tradition. The word 'aya' means life and 'veda' means knowledge in Sanskrit. This medicinal system utilises the laws of nature to bring the body into balance and harmony, working not just on a cellular level but on a much deeper level, treating you physically, emotionally, mentally and spiritually. The mind and body work together to regulate physiology, therefore when a practitioner prescribes medicine, they will also want to prevent illness by balancing the equilibrium of the person's energetic constitution.

Practitioners view the individual as being made up of five elements: ether (space), air, fire, water and earth. When these elements are present in the environment, they will have the same influence on us. Each individual has a direct pattern of energy that defines your characteristics. These are known as our doshas. Every treatment given by the practitioner will have a prescribed protocol based on your basic nature or dosha.

Pitta is made of fire and water. Pitta people are usually of medium frame with warm fair skin and fine hair. They are sharp, intense and determined with intensity in their voice. Pitta people have a good appetite with good digestion and elimination but they need to minimise spicy foods. Pitta people are moderate sleepers. They tend to gravitate more towards cooler conditions.

Vata is made of air and ether. Vata people are usually of a slender frame with prominent joints and delicate dry skin. They are quick and lively in thought and very creative and enthusiastic. Vata people are more suited to warm foods with a heavier texture. They are light sleepers and gravitate towards warmer environments.

Kapha is mostly water with earth. Kapha people have larger frames and have thick skin, tending to oiliness, and thick curly hair. In general they are stable, calm and happy. They crave more pungent, bitter food and have a slower digestion. They have more of a tendency to carry weight and are heavy sleepers. They feel uncomfortable in damp or clammy conditions.

In general we are made of all these three doshas, however at any one time one or two may be more dominant. These doshas can easily be disturbed by stress, unhealthy diet, weather, bad relationships and so on. It is the job of the practitioner to understand which doshas need balancing by carrying out a few simple tests such as asking about your lifestyle, taking your pulse, looking at your tongue, feeling your stomach etc. Using this holistic approach they will advise a diet, yoga and meditation, as well as herbal remedies and treatments.

*Health is wealth. Peace of mind is happiness. Yoga shows the way.*
Swami Vishnu-devananda (1927–93)

# The yogic diet and the triguna

A yogi will eat a vegetarian diet and also have a philosophy based on how much they eat, how the food is prepared and what source the food has derived from. The yogi believes that the foods we consume are a reflection of our characteristics and behaviour, as we are what we eat. These categories of food also determine our behaviour, thinking, health and diet.

▸ Sattvic food, which is the ideal diet of a yogi, would be the most pure in nature and be made from fresh, wholesome, living foods (that is, foods which are grown in direct sunlight). Sattvic people are more balanced, pure and full of vibrancy. They enjoy eating foods that are mild and healthy and are very mindful about what they put into their bodies.

▸ Rajasic food, which has more of a stimulating effect such as caffeine, alcohol, unrefined sugars and spicy foods, can have an effect on our state. Rajasic people are over-stimulated, active, can't sit still and are attached to ego. They enjoy foods which are bitter, sour, salty, hot and spicy.

▸ Tamasic food derives from animals such as meat and dairy products, as well as foods which are fried, stale, processed and decaying or fermented. These are foods which are not conducive to a higher mind as well as causing the body to become susceptible to disease. Tamasic people are more lazy, negative and inert. They suffer from mood swings and are usually self-centred. They eat mindlessly and eat packaged and junk foods. They usually suffer from degenerative disease.

The three characteristics of the gunas, sattva, rajas and tamas, will also be taken into consideration when being analysed by an ayurvedic practitioner.

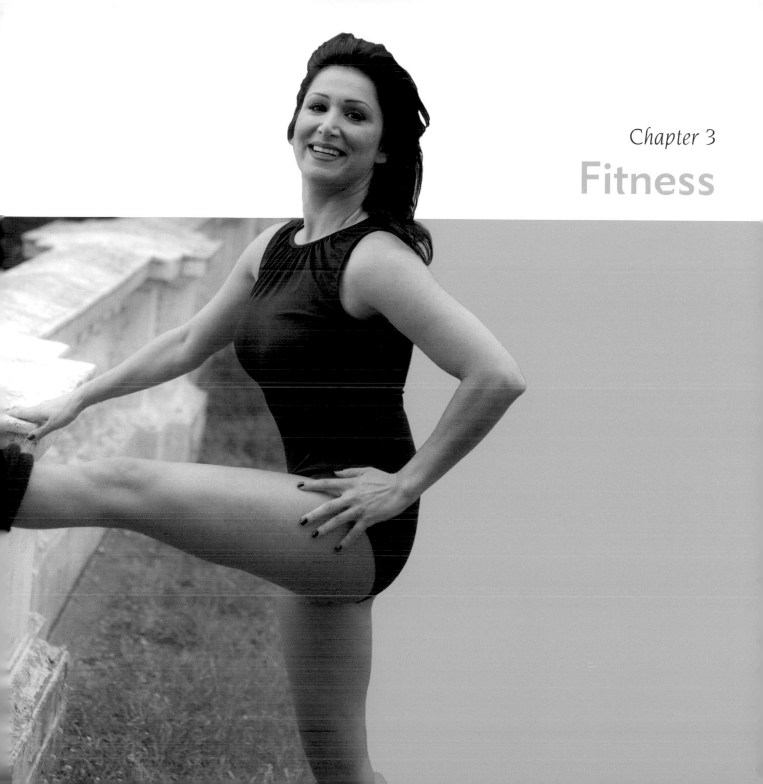

Chapter 3

# Fitness

# Physical Fitness

We have already discussed fitness of the mind, so let us now move on to the physical fitness realm. When you invest in your health, you're really investing in your whole life. There is no other feeling than when you jump out of bed first thing in the morning with an abundance of energy.

I know from my personal experience that when I've stopped exercising for a while (and that hasn't happened very often in 20 years), all my body's functioning systems feel lethargic and my energy becomes deflated instead of vibrant. Personally, I cannot get a good deep sleep and my craving for less nutritious food kicks in. Apart from these effects, I don't seem to bloom with the same kind of vitality and my confidence starts to diminish. Exercise shifts a lot of energy in my physical body. I feel strong physically and mentally. The sensation I experience post work-out is that I have a physical body which feels toned and alive. I literally feel like all the cylinders are firing and ready to go at maximum blast. I even feel my metabolic rate awaken and raring to burn those calories I feed it with. It is no exaggeration to say that my body feels like a super-fuelled machine after a work-out. The sensation of exhilaration and satisfaction is highly recognised by my senses.

This is my high and my experience, however, physiologically I feel like this because of all the changes which occur during and after a work-out.

# Neurotransmitters

One of the explanations of the sensory feelings I have described are due to the fact that the changes which occur through a practice of regular exercise alter your brain chemistry. Your body undergoes neuromuscular, physiological and physical changes in proportion to the amount of exercise you participate in.

First of all, the neurotransmitters, which are natural brain chemicals known for the transmission of information through the body, brain and nerve cells release certain chemicals. One of the main chemicals is serotonin, which is one of the hormones manufactured by the brain. This is well known as the 'happy hormone' because it is a natural mood stabiliser and great for alleviating symptoms of mild depression. Most of the brain cells are influenced by this hormone. During any exercise which involves aerobic activity (any style of cardio-vascular exercise), serotonin levels are elevated and do not revert back immediately post work-out. Serotonin will be released within 30 minutes of activity. However beginners don't need to complete 30 minutes all in one go, this can be broken down into smaller intervals. This 'happy hormone' improves overall feelings of well-being and it helps regulate carbohydrate cravings, sleep cycles and good digestion.

Another neurotransmitter chemical released is norepinephrine which helps to control appetite, emotions and our reaction to stress. Low levels of serotonin and norepinephrine result in depression. People who are physically active are able to recover from depression, control mental health problems and gain a sense of clarity more quickly.

The neurotransmitters also release endorphin and dopamine. Endorphin is released from the pituitary gland (which controls growth and development) into the brain and is known for its painkilling properties. You could say it is the body's natural painkiller as it minimises the discomfort of the pain of exercise. Once the impulses block the pain, frequent exercisers have expressed feeling a euphoric or high sensation afterwards.

Dopamine is a chemical known for its connection with sleep patterns. It has again been associated with cardio-vascular exercise and elevates mainly when serotonin levels are increased. All in all, these 'feel good' chemicals are produced in the body during activity and make a huge difference to the exerciser's energy levels and sense of well-being.

# Health benefits of exercise

There are many health benefits associated with regular exercise, including:

- Heart and blood vessels become stronger
- Improves cardio-vascular fitness
- Improves overall strength and stamina
- Improves memory
- Lifts depression and anxiety
- Reduces blood pressure
- Prevents future disease
- Fights infection
- Promotes a healthy appetite
- Promotes a deep sleep
- Promotes flexibility
- You become fit and agile
- Enhances mood

- Balances body weight
- Changes the whole shape of your body
- Boosts confidence
- Gives you energy
- Oxygenates the whole body to build up a strong immune system
- Speeds up your metabolic rate
- Promotes psychological well-being
- Reduces risk of diabetes and heart disease
- Builds and maintains muscles and joints
- Builds bone density by building bone mineral to prevent osteoporosis
- Prevents weight gain

Again the rewards one can reap from regular exercise are enough to warrant writing a book just on that subject alone. I hope this handful of benefits has given you a great incentive and inspiration to get going. Whenever you feel you're dragging yourself to the gym and not in the mood, get this list out and read it. Even better, photocopy this page and put it up perhaps on your fridge and remember why you keep on track with your training.

# Benefits of having a personal trainer (PT)

We all know that in this day and age a personal trainer is not just for the superstars and extremely wealthy people. In fact, it has become as popular as having your manicure and pedicure. But unless you hire a trainer and gain first-hand experience of how different and much quicker you get results than when exercising on your own, you will never know. In the past I have met my future clients who really were not aware of the vast difference of having a trainer and the transformation it could make to their lives.

When I see individuals training in the gym with limited range, poor posture and clearly a lack of knowledge of which muscle group they are using I am shocked. The most important practice in my world and profession is how you perform your exercises. Whether you are running, doing aerobics or training with resistance the main objective is to be hot on technique, technique and technique. I say this because it is really advisable to have full awareness of your posture when you are training. Using mirrors and understanding how your body works anatomically is of real importance. It is better to do ten repetitions with immaculate posture and good technique than doing 100 sloppy ones. You will reap the benefits of training a lot quicker by avoiding the latter.

It is also better to start with smaller weights if you are strength training and build up your strength before you move onto bigger weights. Struggling with heavy weights and incorrect posture can lead to injury. I also recommend that when you are beginning any type of fitness activity that you build up the time and intensity. Most novices start a training programme with keenness and go crazy within the first few weeks and then drop out as it becomes painful instead of a pleasure. One has to treat it like a lifestyle change and integrate activity gradually into your life. You're not going to sit down in a four-hour-solid crossed-legged lotus position the first time you approach meditation are you? Therefore you have to wean yourself into a regular exercise programme and enjoy each session. Being present in your training sessions instead of rushing to get it over and done with will make a huge difference to your mindset towards exercise.

## Conscious contractions and muscle types

I always make sure my clients are training consciously. Apart from being present one has to apply conscious contractions to every muscle group as you are exercising. In any resistance work where the idea is to change the shape of your body by getting stronger and leaner you will always have a concentric and eccentric action. This means that the muscle you are working is contracting while the counter muscle group is lengthening. An example which most people are familiar with is a bicep curl. When you are doing a bicep curl (front of upper arm) your bicep is contracting and your tricep (back of upper arm) is lengthening. Another name given to this type

of training is agonist and antagonist. When you are doing the bicep curl for instance, this is the time that you apply a conscious contraction to it even if you are using a weight. While performing a bicep curl consciously squeeze your bicep with your own body's force and resistance. Adding a conscious contraction will increase the resistance and make you tone up much faster as well as keep you fully aware of what is happening in your body.

Another great example of a way to apply a conscious contraction is when you are doing a squat. Practise this for a moment. Stand with your legs apart (a little wider than shoulder width). Have your feet slightly turned out and go down into a squat position. Do a few of these and see how it feels. Once you have established the sensation, I want you to consciously turn your attention to the muscles which you feel are weaker when you come up. Naturally, your body will use the strongest muscles and you will not even be aware of this. However, when you come up this time, consciously put all your energy and attention into the inner thighs and use them to lift you as you come up from the squat. This is how you use conscious contractions to your benefit and even out your muscle distribution even better by having full awareness when you are training.

This is what I personally teach my clients. Apart from the fact you are learning about the body and know exactly which muscle group is being engaged, knowing how to get fit and burn fat by using your heart rate are some of the positive reasons for having a trainer.

A trainer will not only educate you but they will become your personal motivator and, hopefully, have the ability to distract you from the pain by cheerleading you on when you're doing the final rep or minute of cardio that you probably wouldn't carry on doing if you were on your own. That last rep or extra five minutes of cardio is what takes you to the next level. Each time you train, ultimately you are increasing your training ability to avoid plateau and maintenance.

I'm also a firm believer in cross-training. This means always chopping and changing your style of work-out in order to shock your muscles and nerve endings so your body doesn't get used to doing the same mundane exercises.

If you are participating in any aerobic activity and not sure whether you are working at about the correct intensity for beneficial purposes, a very basic guideline is the breath test. While you are exercising and over your warm-up section you should be able to speak in short sentences. If you can waffle on, bring the level up or if you cannot speak due to lack of breath, bring the intensity down a notch.

Aerobic exercise and resistance work use different energy pathways. Aerobic/endurance exercise uses your slow-twitch muscle fibres (in long-distance running, cycling and swimming for example). Resistance/strength or any explosive style of training using short, sharp outbursts requires your fast-twitch muscle fibres (for instance in weight training, sprinting and plyometrics).

We all have an even composition of these muscle fibres in our bodies, however, based on our genetic predisposition it is possible for one type of muscle fibre to be slightly more prevalent than another. The ratio of muscular fibres will be dependent on the type of sports activity one participates in. For example, a sprinter would have 75 per cent fast-twitch fibres, whereas the marathon runner would have 75 per cent slow-twitch. Although it is not possible to change these muscle fibre compositions around, one can increase the number of each type of fibre in relation to the specific training genre.

Slow-twitch muscle fibres are usually red in colour. This is because they contain lots of blood vessels which rely on oxygenated blood. Oxygen is required to be utilised for the production of energy in order for the muscle to contract. These muscle fibres contract slowly but can keep going for a long time without getting tired, hence they are connected to any long-distance aerobic activity. The oxygen or air is necessary to breakdown glucose which is the fuel utilised for energy.

Fast-twitch muscle fibres are white in colour and usually thicker. They don't need oxygen to make energy as they use anaerobic (without oxygen) metabolism to create fuel. These fibres fatigue faster as they contract with a much higher velocity consuming lots of energy. Due to the non-use of oxygen a by-product called lactic acid is produced. Lactic acid is a waste product given off in your muscles during anaerobic performance. This waste product will be burned off by your body when it is resting. While the muscles are repairing themselves during the recovery stage they will use oxygen to replenish itself. This is why one should not exercise with weights on the same muscle group consecutively as this doesn't allow enough time for the muscles to go through the biochemical healing process in order for the muscles to grow (hypertrophy). This would be putting the body into overtraining mode and lead to fatigue.

## Convenience

A personal trainer will also be adaptable to fitting in around your lifestyle and schedule. This is very useful for anyone who is time poor and simply cannot make it to the gym. A trainer can come to your home at a suitable time and give you a programme to do at home with minimum equipment that requires very little space. If you're not a gym-lover this can be a real bonus and if you're not a fan of exercise yet need to get healthy for medical reasons it is ideal. Once a trainer rings your doorbell, there is nowhere to hide unless you leave them standing outside in the hope they will disappear! (No chance! They usually show up, rain, hail or snow.)

Having a personal trainer can be a lot of fun (believe it or not) and great for keeping you on track to help meet your target and reach your fitness goals much more quickly, effectively and safely. When a work-out is devised specifically for each individual, the results can be very successful. It can also be versatile depending on where you train. If you work in an office all day, there is nothing better than exercising outside in lovely fresh air.

Not only does it save time having a one-to-one session but it reduces the time needed to achieve results. Each session with a trainer is probably equivalent to three training sessions on your own. As I have mentioned, this way your training will be much more thorough, intense and personalised. Most experienced trainers have great empathy, communication and people skills due to their personal daily interaction with their clients. Therefore you have more than just a knowledgeable teacher watching over you to make sure that you're performing correctly. Basically, you're also recruiting a mentor and a coach who genuinely has an interest in helping you to get healthy.

If having a trainer doesn't fit in with your budget, you can always share a session with a friend to split the price or perhaps cut back on one other hobby or social event. If you look at how often you go out shopping or to dinner, for example, you have to see how much you spend and figure out how much the value of swapping one activity for another that gets you better health is worth to you.

## Types and frequency of exercise

My own personal recommendation of how to exercise is to do cardio (aerobic) exercise three to four times per week for 30–40 minutes. If you don't have so much time for cardio, I would increase the intensity of the exercise each time. For example, if you cut down your cardio time and can only do 20 minutes, which should be the absolute minimum, make sure you are working as hard as you can so you are using up the same energy expenditure as if you were exercising longer. At the end of the day, it's the total calories burned that matters. This way of doing cardio works wonders for your stamina, not to mention that you are still burning calories at a higher rate up to four hours after your work-out.

I would also do strength and resistance work three times per week for 40 minutes or longer. This will totally shape and sculpt your body, especially if you pay attention to your posture and technique. That is a basic sample of the time and frequency. I have found through my personal experience that fitness as a whole energises me physically. When I accompany this with yoga, where I feel the energy is more internal and demands a sense of mind discipline through the breathing, this gives me internal or mental energy, not to mention fantastic flexibility.

The fusion of the two practices is extremely powerful and this is the reason I have created my own personal 'AeroYogaLates' work-out. This is an effective cocktail of the three disciplines. A fantastic work-out for all those who love to practice yoga and aerobic exercise with core work, yet simply have to compensate by doing one or the other due to time restrictions. This work-out will give you outstanding results with the mixture of the three flavours.

## The Fabulous Fitness at 40 work-out

I have personally devised this work-out with the following in mind. First, my main objective is to make sure all the major muscles in the body are fully activated for long-lasting effective results. It really is a top-to-toe, total body conditioning and toning routine to target all the areas. Through regular, consistent practise this work-out will change the shape of your body and make you stronger.

Remember, when you're doing a routine like this, your aim is to create more lean muscle tissue mass in the body instead of having a higher ratio of body fat. This in essence will speed up the metabolic rate as lean muscle tissue is calorie burning. Your muscles will utilise the calories you consume for fuel and energy provided you are active and exercise frequently while building up the intensity. What I mean by the latter is that once you start doing this routine, make sure over time you

increase the repetitions and weight otherwise you will stay at a maintenance level. Unfortunately, this is the big mistake most people make when starting a new fitness regime. They do the same work-out without notching up the level and, of course, after a period of time lose enthusiasm because they are no longer seeing results. I call this the 'plateau stage'.

To avoid this make sure you are constantly challenging yourself and know that after your work-out you are feeling exhilarated, energised and strong. Another common mistake is many people don't make the most of their use of range of motion. This means that when you're performing your exercise, work to a 100 per cent range. If you're doing a shoulder press, for example, and only lift your arms halfway (50 per cent range), you are only going to get 50 per cent results. Be conscious and aware of your posture and technique. As you know already I'm really hot on technique. You know that performing with less heavy weights and great technique will get more successful results, than doing an exercise with heavier weights with poor technique.

Most of the exercises are combinations, meaning you're working two major parts of the body or more at the same time. My special name given to these combination exercises are 'bargain exercises' as in two (or even three if you're lucky) for the price of one.

In this work-out, you will need a set of weights and a mat for the floor-work section. It is not compulsory to start with weights if you're new to exercise. In fact, for beginners, I recommend not using any until you have tried this work-out a minimum of four times. Please remember to give yourself adequate rest from one exercise to the next if it is your first time. If, however, you're a frequent exerciser, I advise starting with 1–2kg (2–4lb) and build up from there to a maximum 4kg (8lb) over a period of time. I will be giving tips of how many repetitions to do depending on your level. You can participate in this work-out three to four times per week to achieve great results.

Remember to stay hydrated throughout your work-out. If you're feeling thirsty, that is your body telling you it is already dehydrated. Drink water, before, during and after working out.

It is very important to breathe when you are performing any exercise. As a general guideline, always exhale on the effort. That is the part which is the most explosive and dynamic. It is the positive work. Inhale on the negative work, that is how you control and release after the effort part of the exercise. The more control you have on the negative work, the better, as there is more time for the nerve endings to send messages to the brain meaning more efficient contractions in the muscle. This means you will tone up quicker due to the controlled action. Rushing your repetitions will not give you the most effective results. This is why it is best to do this work-out to certain beats per minute or follow the DVD.

Remember to use your conscious contractions.

Before you start this routine, unless you are using the DVD, please make sure you warm up. Go for a long power walk or do some stepping up and down and stretches in order to get the heart rate up.

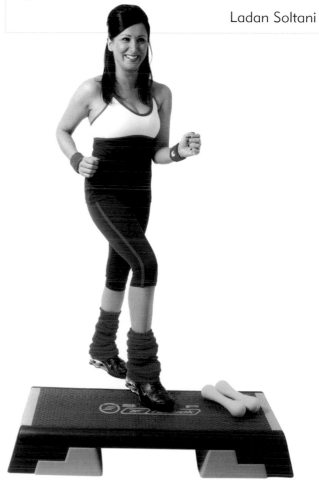

> *The best gift you can give yourself is an investment in your health. To create a happy mind and fit body is priceless yet worth all the wealth in the world.*
>
> Ladan Soltani

*A warm up is the most imperative part of the work-out as it helps minimise injury and maximise performance.*

# THE WORK-OUT

## Exercise 1 alternate lunges and overhead raises

▸ This works the **shoulders** (posterior deltoid) and **legs.**

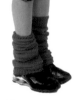

**1** Start by having your feet together and a nice upright posture with the weights resting on your shoulders.

**2** Start lunging forwards with your right leg, keeping the weight centred and making sure your knee does not go forwards over the toes. I always say in lunges that your legs should be at a 90-degree angle on each leg. Make sure that your back heel is lifted off the ground as you stay in this pose and that you are tilting the pelvis forwards.

**3** Now lift the weights overhead into a shoulder press once and step back to the starting position again. Repeat the same thing on the left leg. The combination of stepping forwards and back is four counts, so step forward 1, overhead raise 2, arms back down to shoulders 3, step back 4.

Beginners start with five repetitions on each leg (alternate sides, 10 in total); intermediates do 10 on each leg (alternate sides, 20 in total); and advanced do 10 on the same leg and change sides (20 in total). Intermediates and advanced may repeat the whole exercise by doing it twice through.

# Exercise 2 alternate side lunges and lateral raises

▶ This exercise strengthens and stretches the **inner thighs** and the **shoulders** (medial deltoids).

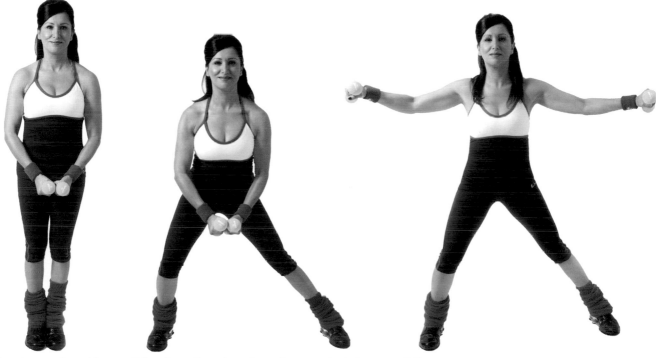

**1** Start by standing with your feet together and arms together in front of the body.

**2** Step laterally to the side, making sure both feet are parallel (facing forward). As you step to the side make sure one leg is fully extended to activate the inner thigh stretch and the other is bent. Keep your posture upright here and avoid leaning too far forward. Most importantly, keep the side lunge within your range so when you come back to the starting position, you feel in control and can step back smoothly and effortlessly.

**3** Do a side lateral raise with your arms, keeping the palms facing downwards and your arms in line with your chest. When you bring the arms back down, bring them back to the centre. Repeat the same exercise to the other side and keep alternating this exercise.

So, the combination is side lunge 1, lateral raise 2, arms back down 3, step together 4.

Beginners start with five repetitions on each leg (alternate sides, 10 in total); intermediates do 10 on each leg (alternate sides, 20 in total), and advanced do 10 on the same leg and change sides (20 in total). Intermediates and advanced may repeat the whole exercise by doing it twice through.

# Exercise 3 squats and forward raises and squats, biceps and outer thigh raises

▸ This exercise works all the **muscles below the belt** and **shoulders** (anterior deltoids) and **biceps**.
The second variation pays more attention to the **outer thighs**.

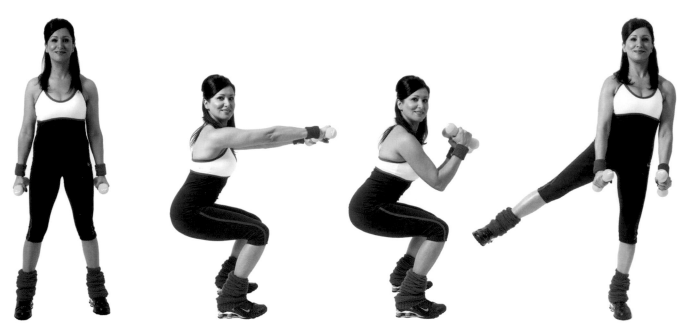

**1** Start by standing with your legs shoulder width apart and your feet facing forward. Make sure that you are aware that the body weight is in your heels.

**2** As you squat, imagine you are sitting back into a chair so that your knees do not come over the toes. As you sit back, keep the stomach muscles fully engaged to support the back. Raise your arms up to the chest with the palms facing downwards as you exhale. Really use the arms to counter-balance the body weight and sit away from them. A very typical mistake on this exercise is that most people have a tendency to lean forward or round the shoulders. Perhaps practise this in front of the mirror so you can see your side profile.

**3** On this exercise do exactly the same squat move, except change the arms to a bicep curl.

**4** As you come up from the squat, lift your outer thigh and avoid leaning to one side to compensate the body weight. Instead use your abdominals to give you good strong support. Repeat this to the other side and keep alternating this move.

Beginners do 10 repetitions of the first variation and 10 each side of the second; intermediates do 20/20, and advanced do 30/30.

# Exercise 4 stationary lunge and single arm chest press

▶ This exercise works all the **major muscles below the belt** and the **chest**. It is a great stabiliser for the **core** and **abdominals**.

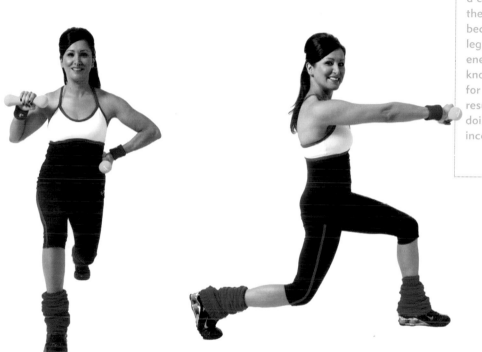

Ladan's lovely lunges can be a challenge for sure. However, they are fantastic and effective because they work all the big leg muscles and use up a lot of energy, and so burn calories. I know when they start to get tough for me, I personally visualise the results in my mind's eye as I'm doing them and this gives me the incentive to keep going!

*Mandy Sydney*

**1** Start In a static lunge. Make sure your body weight is centred and tilt the pelvis under so that your spine is aligned with the back, neck and shoulders.

**2** Use the same arm as the same extended leg, so if you're right leg is leading, use your right arm and place the weight into your armpit with palm facing down. Take the other arm and rest it in your waist.

**3** As you go deeper into the lunge, press your arm forward, keeping it in line with your chest and take it back to the armpit. Keep in the same position and repeat this continuously on the same leg, then change sides.

Beginners do 10 each side; intermediate 20 each side, and advanced 30 each side.

# Exercise 5 rhomboids and rear deltoid raises

▶ This exercise will work the **upper back** and **back of the shoulders**. As you have a stationary posture, it brings great awareness to the control of the **abdomen**. This helps to strengthen the **stomach**. The extended leg will give you a hip flexor stretch and the front leg will be working isometrically. This is a fantastic exercise for anyone who works at a desk all day and needs to improve their posture and make the **thoracic region of the upper body** more lifted and strong.

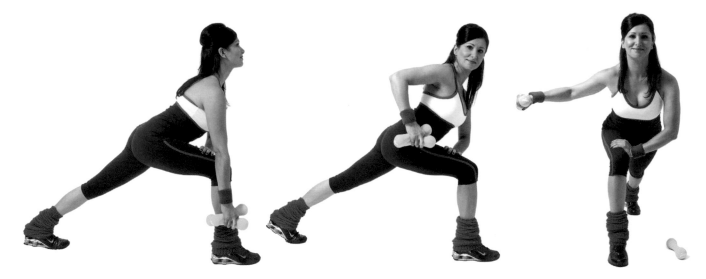

**1** Placing both weights in the same arm as the bent leg, lean forward so that your back is flat and not rounded (you can get this effect by squeezing the shoulder blades together and coming forward from the base of the spine, leading with the chest). Place the opposite hand on the bent leg and let it rest there. Try not to place too much body weight onto the front thigh. Instead, have a strong core to keep supported.

**2** Lift your arm up to a 90-degree angle letting the elbow lead the way, making sure the elbow goes higher than your back and keep the rest of the body completely isolated and still.

**3** This time drop one of the weights and lift your arm laterally to the side bringing the arm no higher than your shoulder.

Beginners do 10 repetitions of the first variation and 10 each side of the second; intermediates do 20/20, and advanced do 30/30.

# Exercise 6 stationary lunge and arm combination

▶ This exercise will work all the **major leg muscles** and is a great **balancing posture**.
It is great for **focusing your mind** and **concentration**, too.

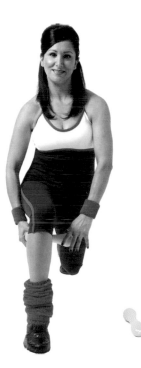

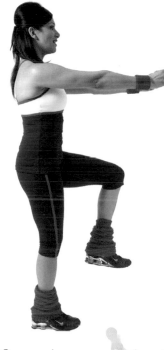

**1** Start in a static lunge position. Whichever leg is leading will have the same accompanying arm. If you start with the right side then place one weight onto that arm and feed it through the outside of the leg. As you feed the weight under the leg, it is really important to pay attention to your posture, making sure you stay upright. Avoid leaning forward by keeping your weight evenly distributed through the centre.

**2** Once you have woven the weight under the leg, bring your arms up to an extended position in front of the body and pull the knee up too. It is now that you have to exhale as you come up and find an unmoveable spot on the floor to help keep your balance. It really helps to activate your core here as posture awareness is a must.

Once you have completed this exercise on one leg, change and repeat on the other side.

Beginners do 10 repetitions each side; intermediates 20, and advanced 30.

# Exercise 7 stationary lunge with rear thigh raise and chest raise

▶ This exercise is great for counter-balancing the body weight and working **legs**, **glutes** (bottom) and **chest**. It is a great exercise for **co-ordination**, **control** and having **awareness of the core**.

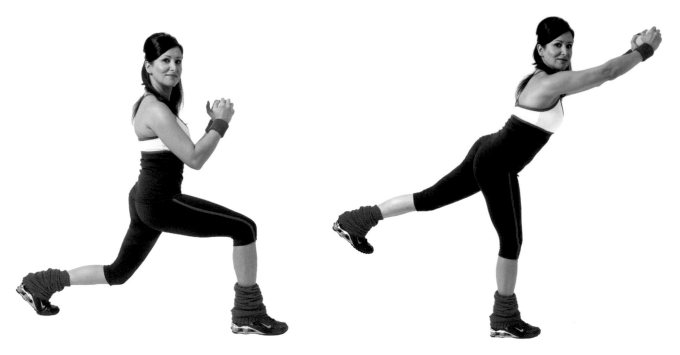

**1** Start by lunging back on one leg, making sure your front leg does not go forward over the toes. Hold one weight in both hands and keep the abdominal muscles pulled in.

**2** As you exhale, extend the arms and legs away from one another, lifting the back leg without arching the lower back. Scoop your arms up by consciously squeezing the chest and have the palms facing upwards going overhead but not fully extended. Repeat this to the other side.

Beginners do 10 repetitions on each side; intermediates 20, and advanced 30.

# Exercise 8 reverse triceps

▶ This exercise will work the **back of your arms**. If you want to wear short sleeves for the rest of your life then this is the one exercise that will do the trick. Women especially have a tendency to carry fat in this part of their body and unless you work it regularly, the appearance of the skin can become very saggy, hence the name 'bingo wings'.

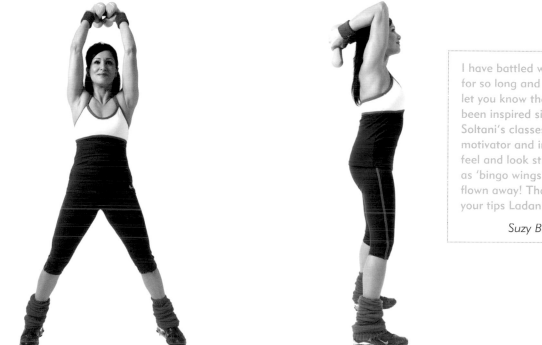

I have battled with my arms for so long and I just want to let you know that I have really been inspired since doing Ladan Soltani's classes. She is a great motivator and inspirer. My arms feel and look strong and as far as 'bingo wings' go, mine have flown away! Thanks so much for your tips Ladan! Simply brilliant.

*Suzy Batton, London, UK*

**1** Start with a good strong posture. Take the legs slightly apart and micro bend the knees to take any tension away from the lower back. Tilt the pelvis forward and keep your stomach engaged. Bring the arms up and glue your arms by your ears ('keep your ears warm'). Keep both weights even and pressed together.

**2** Start to bend the arms from the elbows down, keeping the upper arm still. The closer you keep the upper arms by your ears and isolate them, the more effective are the results on the triceps.

Keep doing this exercise to the point of failure (until you feel you cannot physically do anymore) and drop one of the weights and repeat with just one weight. Once you have exhausted your arms with one weight, try this with only applying your own body weight. Press the palms together to create tension in the arms and repeat the same triceps exercise. This method is called 'drop set', where you are decreasing the weight and depleting the muscle of all its energy.

All levels do two sets of maximum effort using the technique above.

# Exercise 9 standing alternate waist

▶ This exercise works your **sides**, loosening your **lower back** and giving you **mobility** and **flexibility**, as well as **toning around the midriff**.

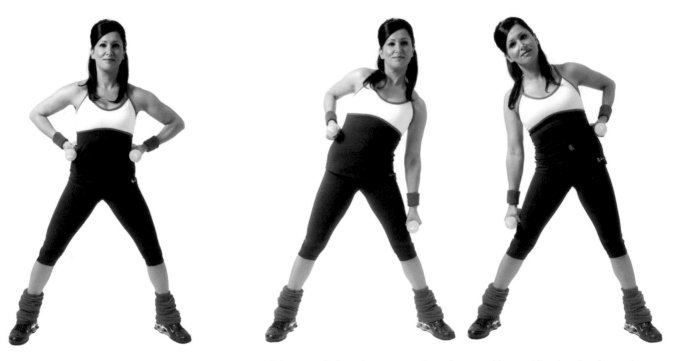

**1** Start by standing with your legs apart, feet pointing at ten and two o'clock. Tilt the pelvis under and micro-bend the knees. Pay attention to the stomach muscles. Even though you're going to be working the waist, you must focus on keeping the stomach pulled in and clenching your glutes (bottom). Place both arms into your waist and make sure that your arms always come back to this point.

**2** As you exhale, take one arm down by your side, avoiding leaning forward. As you do this exercise more and your back loosens up, try to aim to bring the side stretch further each time you do it, aiming to bring the weight below the knee.

Beginners do 20 alternate each side for two sets; intermediates 30 alternate each side for two sets, and advanced 40 alternate each side for two sets.

# Exercise 10 lying down single arm chest flys

▶ Floor work (please use a mat). This exercise will be a great stabiliser for activating the **core** and working the **chest muscles**.

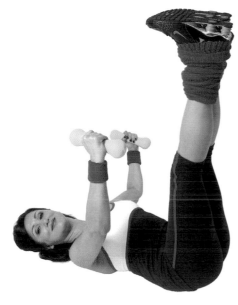 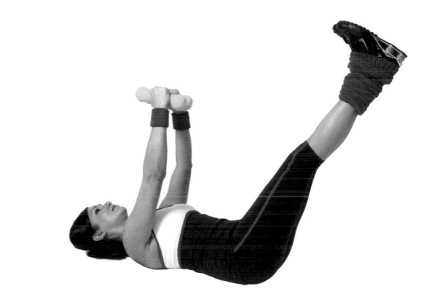

**1A** Lying down on your back in a supine position, bring both legs up in the air to create a 90-degree angle. You have to really keep the stomach muscles tight to keep your legs in that position. Think about pulling the stomach in internally, glueing your lower back into the floor. Flex your feet and have the legs active and straight. Start the arm positioning by making sure both weights are mirroring you.

**1B - Advanced version only** Start by taking one arm down at a time, slightly bending the elbow and stopping the arm from touching the floor. The whole point of this exercise is to keep the core engaged and centred to avoid leaning the body towards the direction of the arm as it goes down. Make sure you do this on an alternate arm.

Next time you're working out and that voice in your head tells you to stop because you're tired, reprogram your way of thinking by visualising the results. Know exactly how reaching your goal will make you feel – at the end of the day, how badly do you want it?

Beginners do 10 repetitions each side and repeat for two sets; intermediates do 20 each side and repeat for two sets.
Advanced do the same repetitions as intermediate, however, take the legs further away from the body to make the intensity around the core region more challenging. The most important point is to remember to close the gap between the mat and your lower back.

# Exercise 11 lying down outer thigh exercise

▶ This is a great exercise for working and toning the **outer thighs** and **hips**. It really is one for targeting and 'hitting the spot'.

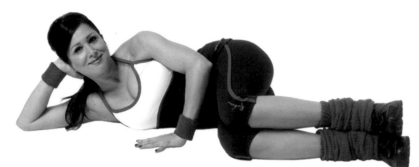

**1** Lie down on your side and bring both legs to a 90-degree angle. Rest your head in the palm of your hand on your elbow and bring the other arm down on the floor in front of your chest.

> After I do Ladan's class, I can vouch that this 'hot hip' exercise (as she calls it) really works wonders on my thighs. Thanks to Ladan, I have dropped two clothes sizes since following her classes and her healthy eating plan. I feel very pleased and excited that I can finally buy the outfits I had only dreamed of wearing.
>
> *Pamela Stoke, Kent*

**2** Extend the outer leg fully and bring it towards your navel. Flex the foot and have the toes pointing towards the floor and the heel towards the ceiling. Start to lift the leg up and down without leaning backwards and keep the stomach engaged.

Exhale as you lift the leg.

A common mistake is rolling backwards as you raise the leg, to make sure you don't, only lift the leg slightly higher than the hip.

Repeat this exercise to the other side.

### Ladan's tip

*Ladies, is it 'hot hips' or 'hot chips'? Which do you prefer?*

Beginners do 20 repetitions each side; intermediates 30 repetitions for two sets, and advanced do 30 repetitions for three sets, or do two sets using ankle weights.

# Exercise 12 inner thigh raises

▶ This exercise speaks for itself and so do the results.

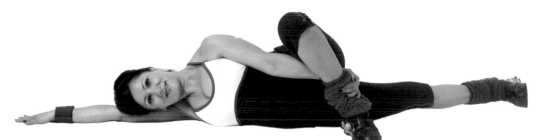

**1** Lie down on your side and bend the outside leg up the body as high as you can so your heel is fully grounded. Take the same arm as this leg and grab your ankle by feeding your hand on the inside of the leg. Lie down completely flat with your upper body keeping the whole body in a straight line.

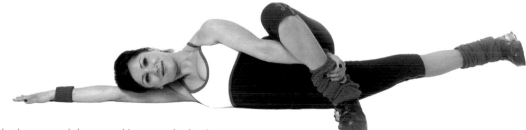

**2** Start to lift the leg up and down, making sure the leg is fully active and extended. Flex your foot a little so that your heel is leading the way. Keep the whole leg in line with the rest of the body and avoid touching the ground as you take the leg down. Make sure you exhale as you lift the leg. Repeat again on the other side.

Beginners do 20 repetitions each side; intermediates 20 repetitions each side for two sets, and advanced 30 repetitions each side for three sets, or do two sets using ankle weights.

# Exercise 13 rear thigh raises

▶ This is a great exercise for building a **high, perky bottom** and hopefully keeping it there. Also a great **core** exercise.

**1** Start by going onto your elbows and knees. Lift one leg up letting the heel lead the way and face the ceiling. Keep your hands located under your chest and avoid leaning too far forward. The most important point in this exercise is to keep the stomach fully engaged even though you're breathing. Make sure the lower back does not arch either way. By being aware of the abdominals you create an even, neutral spine throughout.

**2** Point the knee down to the opposite heel making sure the knee goes over the top of the heel. Again pay attention to your posture, keeping the rest of the body still as you do this movement.

Beginners do 20 repetitions each side; intermediates 20 repetitions each side for two sets, and advanced 30 repetitions each side for three sets, or do two sets using ankle weights.

# Exercise 14 abdominal section and core stability

▶ These exercises are going to work your **stomach**, **obliques** and **back**.

## Abdominal 1

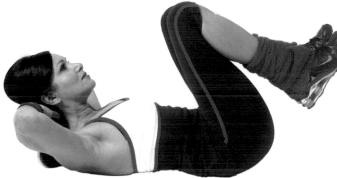

**1** Lying on your back, bring your knees into your chest and arms behind your head to support it.

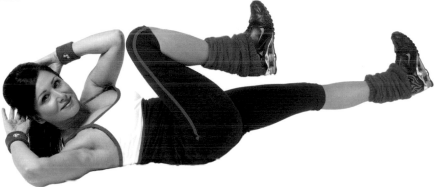

**2** Alternate your opposite elbow to knee making a cycling action. The most important point is to keep your lower back glued into the mat. If your back is arching, then I suggest you don't extend the levers so far out. Initially keep the knees closer to the body until your stomach muscles and back feels stronger. Try not to twist so much by keeping in control and balancing your body weight more centrally.

Beginners do 10 repetitions for two sets, keep the knees bent and do not take them far away from the body; intermediates do 20 repetitions for two sets, you can explore by taking the legs as far as is safe for you, and advanced do 30 repetitions for two sets, again exploring by taking the legs as far as is safe for you.

# Exercise 14 (continued)

## Abdominal 2

**1** On this exercise, you're going to extend your legs fully and rest your heel on top of your toe, keeping the legs very active. Make sure you close the gap between your lower back and the ground.

**2** As you are doing this sit-up, make sure your head stays in line with your spine so that you're not using your neck by pushing it forward when you come up and down. Also consciously contract the stomach muscles as you come up and keep them contracted on the way down even though you are breathing. In these exercises, exhale as you come up. Please remember, you only need a 45-degree lift for your stomach muscles to be fully contracted. If you come up beyond that point, you engage the hip flexors and the lower back.

One arm is fully extended, while the other arm is gripping the extended arm to make a head-rest or pillow for your head.

Beginners take the conventional sit-up arm position to start with (both arms behind head). Also bend your legs in slightly to keep the lower back supported.

# Stretching exercises

When you are stretching, your receptors on the nerve endings send messages to the brain that you are stretching a specific muscle. This process takes about 6–8 seconds to register, so please be patient with holding them and after a while increase the stretch by breathing deeply. Stretching at the end of the work-out is hugely beneficial and highly recommended. It will help to produce greater mobility, flexibility and range of motion, as well as decreasing a build-up of waste products given off in your muscle during the contraction phase of an exercise.

## Abdominal stretch

Keep the hands and hips grounded. Take the shoulders away from the ears by squeezing back the shoulder blades.

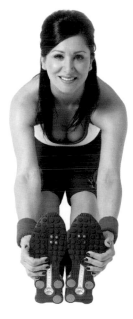

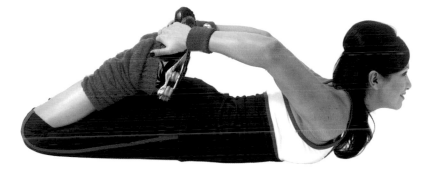

## Hamstring stretch

As you're coming forward, make sure your chest is leading the way and you're coming down from the base of your spine, keeping the legs as active as possible and the feet flexed.

## Quadriceps stretch

Bring your heels to your bottom and grab hold of the ankles. Beginners may do it lying on one side and do one leg at a time.

**Note:** please don't hold your breath on any of the stretches.

# Stretching exercises (continued)

## Standing hip flexor and chest stretch

Stand in a static lunge position and really tilt the pelvis forward to stretch the hip flexor. Interlace your arms behind your back and squeeze the shoulder blades together, opening up the chest…

… change sides and do exactly the same as the previous exercise but change the arms to a shoulder stretch, interlacing your arms so the palms are facing upwards.

## Thigh and hip stretch

Sitting nice and tall, cross one leg over the other and give it a nice big hug. Make sure your posture remains upright.

# Stretching exercises (continued)

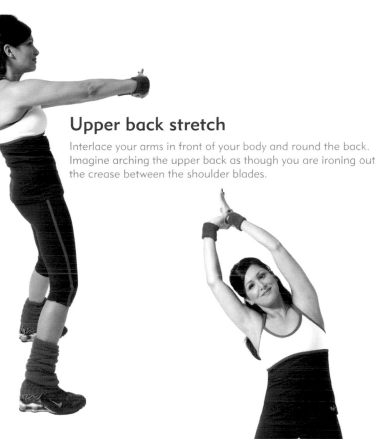

## Upper back stretch

Interlace your arms in front of your body and round the back. Imagine arching the upper back as though you are ironing out the crease between the shoulder blades.

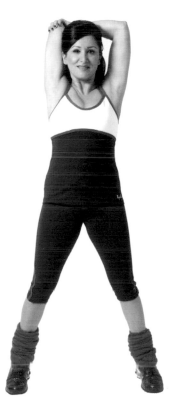

## Triceps stretch

Take one arm behind to the opposite shoulder and take the opposite arm to the top of the elbow and gently resist by pulling the elbow back.

## Side stretch

Stand with your legs wide and grab hold of one wrist with one arm and stretch the body to one side making sure you do not push your hip out. Avoid leaning forwards and don't bend the knee on the same side of the waist that you're stretching to compensate. Do this on each side.

'No pain, no gain? Not in my world. Just dedicate your work-out to someone you love and trust me, there will be no pain, only pleasure!

Ladan Soltani

That brings us to the end of the work-out. I hope you had fun doing this and the best advice I can give is to persevere. Once you start to see results, this will naturally motivate you to keep going. Remember, exercising the physical body is the same as exercising the mind. In fact they really go hand in hand and need to be a part of your lifestyle. There is no 'quick fix' if you want it for the long term. If you want to keep the results, expect to take a period of time to build this up, starting by creating a foundation of a really strong, toned body. Once you become a regular exerciser, you will find that when you stop for a short while, then return to exercising again, it will never be like the first time you trained as your muscles have memory and react to stimulation instantly.

To keep motivated to keep going, I have a list of suggestions of what you may do to stay focused and positive so that you stick to your regime. I also include other ways of keeping fit and healthy, without necessarily having to do a conventional work-out if you're looking for a change.

## 20 motivational ideas to keep on exercising

1   Choose an exercise style which you really enjoy. Remember, make your work-out a fun, joyful event so you look forward to your sessions.

2   If you're not good at staying motivated, find a partner to train with or make it a social event where a bunch of your friends all work out together. This will always be a great way to get you going on the days you feel less inspired as you can become each other's cheerleader.

3   Hire a professional personal trainer and in making this commitment to yourself and your trainer this will give you the incentive to keep going because you'll have a motivator supporting you during your work-out.

4   If you work better with goal setting, make a plan of how you want to look by a certain date. Remember to use your visualisation techniques and have a picture ready of how you'd like your body to be in a certain time frame. Give yourself a target every week and decide how much trimmer and fitter you're going to look.

5   If you love the great outdoors, find an exercise suitable such as power walking or running outside instead of a treadmill indoors. Also these days there are lots of walking and running clubs you can join which are very reasonably priced. You can even set up your own one with a group of friends.

6   How about meeting your friends and going rollerblading or even ice skating instead of dinner or coffee and cakes?

7   Arrange to have a home visit from a fitness professional who can show you how to utilise the furniture in your own home for a work-out.

8   Cycle to work instead of using public transport.

9   Use stairs whenever you can. Believe it or not, I had a friend who used to have a showroom which was on two floors. She never had lifts or elevators in the building. Eventually she moved premises and her new office was on one floor only. She actually gained pounds due to a lack of activity by no longer being able to use the stairs.

10 Go dancing with your friends after a heavy meal and burn off the calories or, if it is a nice evening, go for a stroll and expend a little energy.

11 Drink tons of water when you're sitting at your desk so you have to keep getting up to go to the toilet and burn extra calories.

12 Do a bathroom work-out and dance while brushing your teeth and get a little exercise at the start of your day.

13 Sitting on a swiss ball at your desk will not only improve your posture but it will make you sit properly, engaging your core muscles and making your stomach and back stronger. If you do this, start with short periods and build up your time.

14 Go window shopping at lunchtime and wear a rucksack with a small weight in your backpack to expend more calories than usual. Carry any shopping bags evenly on both arms as you walk fast back to work and do some arms raises with them to get the heart rate up.

15 If you're at home exercising on a treadmill, put on your favourite TV soap to keep you distracted.

16 If you have a dog, take it for interval runs in the park and time yourself to do one minute of running/walking. Also you can use the park bench to do a variety of strength training exercises such as press-ups and tricep dips (works chest muscles and backs of arms).

17 If you're a yummy mummy and want to burn the baby fat, I suggest buying a style of pram which enables you to do a brisk power walk or light jogging intervals. The best way to diminish the excess weight of pregnancy is to nip it in the bud within the first 12 months while you have all the extra hormones in the body to help you heal and recover.

18 Walk everywhere when possible.

19 Massage your partner to burn extra calories.

20 Always keep a picture of how you want to look in your mind's eye, especially when it comes to running that last mile or lifting the last repetition. This will make you stronger mentally and help you resist that dessert.

These are a few simple ideas to motivate you to start. I find once I make a habit of doing some of the above on a regular basis that it becomes a part of my life and something I can't live without.

Plan your work-out sessions in advance and make a point of writing them in your diary. To succeed you need to find something to focus on which you enjoy. It should never feel like a chore when you're working towards achieving it.

Sometimes you have to step a little out of your comfort zone and take that extra inch. Anyone who achieved something out of the ordinary never stayed within the realms of their comfort. Go for it. Program the subconscious mind to make it work for you and to make it all happen because you deserve to give yourself the body you desire.

*The future is not set in stone, it is your actions which govern the next pages of your story.*

Charlie Mould

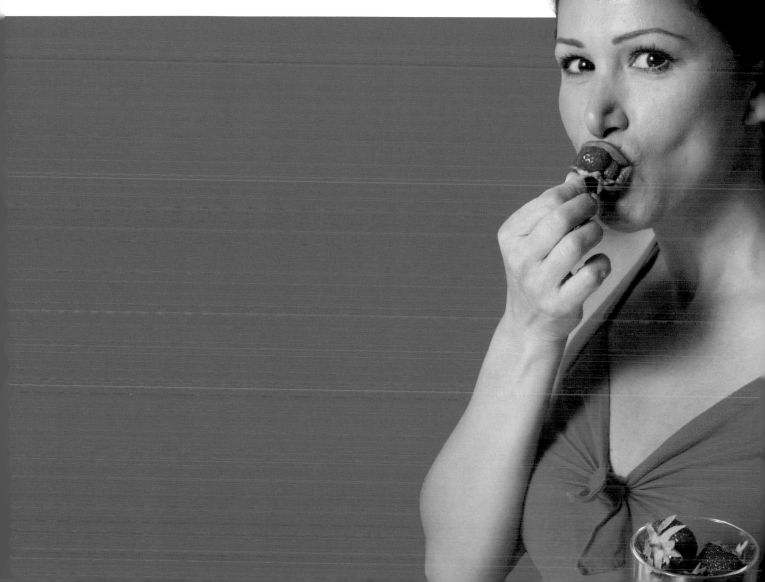

# Chapter 4

# Diet and Nutrition

# Getting the balance right

This subject is controversial and vast. I believe each individual's body is unique, due to many influences including gender, constitution, character and emotions, to name but a few. If we become more mindful and aware of the body's nutritional needs, it tells us what we should eat. There is no doubt that diet is probably the most important factor for losing weight in order to keep it off.

Let's put it this way, if you are exercising regularly, doing everything by the book yet not losing weight, then you really have to address your diet. It's no secret that if your calorie consumption is higher than your levels of energy expenditure your answer is weight gain – regardless of how much time you are spending in the gym.

I recommend eating small, regular meals to sustain your blood sugar levels and to keep that metabolic rate stimulated. Breakfast is very important as this is the time of the day that your blood sugar levels are at their lowest and need a good boost for balance. You will definitely find that if you fuel up first thing in the morning you're less likely to have cravings in the evenings. For healthy snacks between meals or prior to training, I would choose foods that are a mixture of carbohydrates and protein such as fruit and nuts, or a slice of wholemeal bread with peanut butter (ideally organic).

Smoothies are also a great source of instant energy for pre/post training or as a meal replacement. A great all-round smoothie is one that has some form of protein, fruit, natural yogurt or soya milk with nuts and seeds. It will give you a great booster for energy before your work-out as it will dissolve into the bloodstream quicker than if you had to break food down by chewing. I have created a few recipes of my own and will share these with you (see page 112).

Getting the right balance of nutritional calories from your food is key and vital for acquiring sufficient vitamins and minerals to give your body the correct diet.

# Exercise and diet

These two subjects really go hand in hand. It's not the latest news that when you start to work out your body naturally starts craving healthier food. As you become fitter your whole constitution changes and your liver gets a good cleanse from all the extra water you're drinking as well as the intake of more oxygen. All of the bodily functions are affected and stimulated positively.

Most people notice that their alcohol intake drops as they cannot handle drinking as many units as before. You become more health conscious and eat more conscientiously. Eating correctly to provide optimum fuel for exercise is imperative.

It is not uncommon to think that only exercise will help you achieve all your fitness goals but food has a huge role to play and really is the major factor. On the other hand, it is wrong to assume that by dieting alone, your body will look aesthetically more shapely. If you lose weight through only diet and shed a lot of pounds, your skin and tissues will not look tight, toned and lean. These two disciplines really operate in union to give you the ultimate results.

# How should I eat and exercise?

The main source of fuel for exercise is carbohydrates. Carbohydrates come in two forms, simple and complex. Simple carbs dissolve quicker into your bloodstream and complex are more slow to release.

Foods such as wholemeal bread, pasta, brown rice, potato and certain vegetables (root) are considered complex carbs, whereas foods such as bananas, dried fruit, cereal, honey, milk, chocolate, cakes, cookies etc are considered simple carbs.

Whichever style of exercise you have adopted, carbohydrates are the energy providers. Once you consume foods which contain carbs, it is broken down in your body into smaller sugars. If it is not used up for energy straight away, it will be stored in your muscles and liver in the form of glycogen. Glycogen is a source of fuel which is easily accessible for any exercise activity. It will always be utilised as fuel whether your exercise involves the slow-twitch or fast-twitch energy pathway. If you don't use up the stored glycogen as energy, it will get stored as fat.

If your body is not loaded with sufficient carbohydrate stores while exercising, your body will resort to other sources to provide energy, such as protein, putting your body into a catabolic state (destructive metabolism). Protein is broken down into a long chain of amino acids (20). In fact, most of your body's functions are reliant on protein.

Ideally, your aim is not to break down the protein as it is required as the building blocks in your body to help repair and maintain your tissues, such as muscle, bone, skin and hair. This is why it is advised to fuel up before a work-out but eat lightly if less than an hour before. Have your main carb and protein meal within the first 60 minutes of a strenuous work-out to replenish glycogen stores and aid in the healing and repair of the muscle tissue. This will also instantly energise your body and sustain your blood sugar and stop you from feeling fatigue.

Examples of protein foods are meat, fish, seafood, eggs, milk, cheese, yogurt, dairy products, nuts, seeds, beans, pulses and certain vegetables.

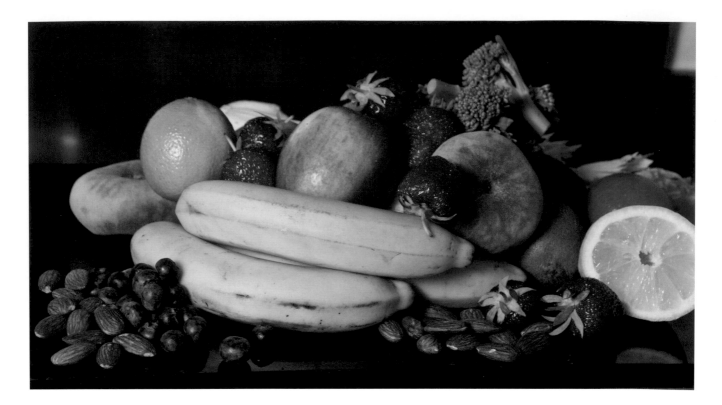

# GI diet and eating for weight-loss

What is the GI diet and how can it help with weight loss? All carbohydrates have a glycaemic index (GI) but some foods may be higher in GI than others. This is to do with how the carbohydrates affect our blood sugar levels when they are broken down into our bloodstream after we consume them.

Low GI foods slowly release sugar into the blood providing a stable balance of energy, which makes you feel full up and satisfied. High GI foods inject a surge of sugar, raising blood sugar levels, which invariably leaves you craving another dose shortly after.

When you consume carbohydrates, it gets broken down into glucose in your body. Your pancreas will secrete a hormone called insulin to break down and carry the sugar from your bloodstream into your cells to be used as energy. If you eat a high sugary food, your body panics and wants to get the blood sugar regulated so it will produce even more insulin than normal to bring the blood sugar down to its natural state. However, because of this, blood sugar levels plummet to lower than their original state, leaving you craving more sugary foods. As high GI foods are quicker to break down and create a rapid rise followed by a drop in blood sugar levels, this leads to eating more often and produces an insulin flood in your system. If you eat lots of these foods, chances are you're more likely to store excess fat because insulin makes you store fat if there is too much sugar in your blood.

# Examples of GI foods

| | LOW GI FOODS<br>55 or less | MEDIUM GI FOODS<br>56–69 | HIGH GI FOODS<br>70 or more |
|---|---|---|---|
| Cereals | Special K 54, All bran 51<br>Oatmeal 49 | Weetabix 69 | Cornflakes 84<br>Rice krispies 82 |
| Breads | Pumpernickel bread 51 | Wholemeal bread 69<br>Pitta bread 57 | Baguette 95, Bagel 72<br>White bread 70 |
| Rice/pasta | Brown rice 50,<br>Macaroni 45, Noodles 40<br>Wholemeal spaghetti 37<br>Fettucine 32 | White spaghetti 67<br>Basmati rice 58 | Steamed rice 98 |
| Fruit | Banana 55, Orange 44<br>Grapes 46, Plum 39<br>Apple 38, Grapefruit 25 | | |
| Vegetables | Corn 55, Carrots 49<br>Broccoli 10, Onion 10<br>Lettuce 10, Mushrooms 10<br>Red pepper 10 | | Parsnip 97, Baked potato 93<br>Boiled potato 70 |
| Dairy | Skimmed milk 32, Low-fat yoghurt 33<br>Whole-milk 22 | Whole-fat ice cream 61 | |
| Beans | Baked beans 48, Lentils 30<br>Chickpeas 28, Kidney beans 27<br>Peas 22, Soyabeans 18 | | Broad beans 79 |
| Snacks | Popcorn 55, Chocolate bar 49<br>Dried apricots 31, Cashews 22<br>Walnuts 15, Peanuts 14 | Ryvita 69 | Rice cakes 82, Cornchips 72 |

These values are taken from the GI Index (www.glycemicindex.com)

# Fats

There is a big misconception that fats make you fat. This is not the case. First, not all fats are bad for you. We need certain natural sources of fat in our body to protect our organs, use for energy and for specific fat-absorbing vitamins.

Fats are made up of molecules called fatty acids, which are either saturated, unsaturated or mono/polyunsaturated. Animal fats (red meat, dairy, eggs and fried foods, etc) are associated with saturated fat and are fats which are solid at room temperature. We should eat this type of fat in moderation. These fats can block up your arteries and build up cholesterol, producing more LDL (low-density lipoprotein). When you exercise, you produce more HDL (high-density lipoprotein), which eats up the LDL and dilates and unclogs the arteries.

The main bad fats to avoid are transfats, otherwise known as hydrogenated fat. This type of fat undergoes a chemical process to change the consistency from turning oil into solid fat. This is called hydrogenation. This synthetic, artificial process change serves no purpose to a health-conscious person who is aware of what they are putting into their body.

If you're being careful about your weight and want to eat healthily, always check the labels on your food.

Good fats are those that have a health benefit and these are monounsaturated and polyunsaturated. These fatty acids, such as nuts, seeds, oils, avocados and oily fish are high in omega 3, 6 and 9. Good fats can help reduce cholesterol. They are also required to prevent heart disease, arthritis and to help a healthy functioning immune system. A balanced regular dose of these fats is also great for balancing hormones and emotions and promoting healthy skin and hair. The anti-inflammatory properties found in these good fats are known for reduction in joint pain and healthier digestion.

When consuming carbohydrates, proteins and fats you need a balance of all three. As a general guideline for someone who is regularly exercising, I recommend 60 per cent of your diet to be carbohydrates, 20 per cent protein and 20 per cent fat (essentially good fats). Each gram of carbohydrate and protein is equivalent to four calories and each gram of fat is nine calories.

# Acid and alkaline body

To restore and maintain good health our blood needs to be slightly alkaline. In order to maintain a healthy PH balance an alkaline diet is highly recommended. The body's PH balance is about 7.35–7.45. If you're below 7.00 PH your body is too acidic.

If you are eating a diet which generates acidity in your body, your immune system will become a magnet for sickness and poor health. Human blood should be slightly alkaline to prevent over acidification in our bodies known as acidosis. Foods which are acidic, such as animal products, sugar, chocolate, wheat, caffeine, yeast and carbonated drinks decrease the body's ability to absorb minerals and reduce the energy production in cells, which makes it harder to

repair damaged cells. An over-acidic system also changes the mineral composition of the cells, which can be corrected by rebalancing the sodium and potassium element.

If you eat a diet of alkaline foods such as greens, vegetables, fruit, beans, lentils, seeds and nuts, this will help your body fight to neutralise the excessive acid in your bloodstream and regenerate the cells. Once this acid is eliminated, fat remaining in the body is no longer required to store acid waste so there is no need for new fat cells to be formed. You will feel the difference in your body after this.

Ideally, 80 per cent of your diet should be from alkaline-producing foods and 20 per cent acid-producing foods.

This is also why it is essential to drink plenty of water while exercising. If you're working the fast-twitch muscle fibres and producing lactic acid (the waste product given off in your muscles), you need to keep your body fuelled with water in order to flush out all the waste and neutralise the acid state. This will also help reduce muscle soreness.

# Wheatgrass

I have to give wheatgrass a huge dedication and mention here as I swear by this product. Wheatgrass is the young grass of the wheat plant that is juiced or dried into powder form. The beneficial properties of wheatgrass are immeasurable, hence it has been given the name superfood.

First of all, it has an abundance of alkaline minerals and there is no wheat or gluten in wheatgrass. It is a vegetable that has sprouted from the seed, however not yet produced a seed itself.

Wheatgrass is mainly known for the high amount of chlorophyll it contains, which is classified as the blood of the plants pigment. Chlorophyll strengthens the cells and detoxifies the liver. It also helps break down chemicals and pollutants in the body.

All in all, wheatgrass will supply you with the most important vitamins, minerals and enzymes and 17 out of the 20 amino acids. It is a fantastic immune booster and great for vegetarians or vegans who need a high protein substitute.

One ounce of wheatgrass is equivalent to two gallons of milk. If you think about it, if you're calcium deficient, why would you drink milk which is being consumed through a second-hand recycled process? We can go directly to the source and get all our requirements instantly without the chemical processes to produce milk.

Other benefits of wheatgrass are that it cleanses and eliminates toxins in the body including heavy metals. It is a great resource for calcium, magnesium and potassium. It will improve digestion and aid in balancing blood sugars to curb sweet cravings. Overall wheatgrass heals the body internally.

Wheatgrass has become more widely recognised as people have become more health-conscious and interested in the nutritional content of the foods they are consuming.

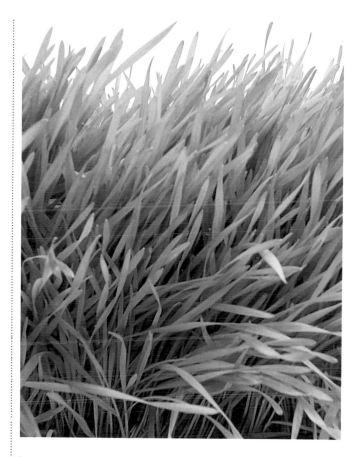

It may be an acquired taste, however, personally I think it is a very small price to pay for the amazing health benefits it provides. I have provided my own smoothie recipe with wheatgrass for anyone who really wants to blend the funky taste if you have sensitive taste buds (see page 114).

# Water

Water is the essence of life and the most important ingredient after oxygen for survival. Every living organism needs water to survive. Over half of your body is made up of water; this mineral plays a vital role in nearly every bodily function. Water also carries oxygen to the cells and protects your organs and joints.

We need water to regulate our body temperature and for the transportation of nutrients to all our organs and waste elimination.

It is very important to stay hydrated and drink even more if we are involved in any sport activity. Lack of hydration can lead to imbalance, weakness of the immune system and it keeps the body in an acidic state. When you're dehydrated you will develop headaches, fatigue and lack concentration. It will also make the kidneys work overtime to eliminate waste products. Always keep hydrated by drinking only water. You will receive 20 per cent of water from food and other beverages, however, no other source will give you the health benefits of drinking pure water alone. Aim to drink 1.5–2 litres a day (3–4 pints) and drink more if you're in a hot climate or exercising as you will be perspiring even more.

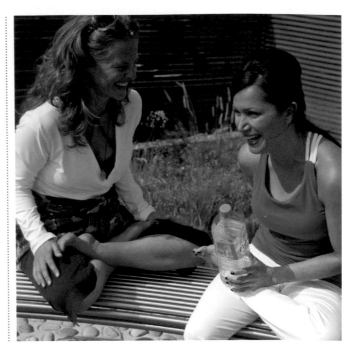

# Water heals

Water has magical healing qualities too. Masau Emoto, a Japanese author and entrepreneur, discovered that if you talk to water or expose it to sounds and music it can change its molecular structure because it has memory.

Once you expose water to harmonious sounds or words, you freeze the water overnight and this is when the crystal formation will take place. When you examine the water crystals under a microscope the aesthetic structures are either beautiful or ugly depending on what the water was exposed to. If you feed it with negative words and energy, the water crystals form shapes similar to the cells of cancer. If you feed it with positive words and beautiful sounds, the crystals form

beautiful diamond-shaped patterns. If you then use this water to drink, you would be transmitting all this information to each and every cell in your body. As you know, water transports oxygen to the cells. If most of your body is made up of water and your muscles have memory, then this is a great holistic way to heal yourself naturally.

# Unhealthy eating patterns

Unhealthy eating patterns can lead to an eating disorder. An eating disorder or an unhealthy eating pattern occurs when an individual's approach to food and body image changes and becomes almost obsessive, unmanageable, leaving huge potential for causing damage to health. This usually stems from feelings of low self-esteem and self-worth.

It is not just women who suffer from this, however a bigger proportion of women go through an eating disorder at some point in their lives.

Social, media and emotional factors can contribute to an eating disorder. Poor self-image is a symptom. The individual may see themselves completely differently to how others see them.

Having gone through my own personal experience of unhealthy eating habits, I understand that there is a thin line to draw in knowing how to set the boundaries with food. Unlike other compulsions and addictions, which can be totally eliminated from one's life, one cannot abstain from eating altogether. It is about understanding where to create boundaries which do not overlap into emotional eating which inevitably becomes habitual.

There seems to be a big correlation with the types of food choices one craves when using food as a way to soothe, comfort and numb one's feelings. I found sugar to be my most-wanted food. Put it this way, when you want to gorge on food knowing that you're not hungry and it is beyond eating for pleasure, you're not exactly going to cry out for broccoli are you? I think a good starting point whether you're under- or over-eating is to keep a thorough food and emotions diary. It may come as a surprise and you may notice a pattern of when you eat food which is triggered by emotion. I suggest keeping a diary for at least one month and be honest, literally writing everything down that you're eating along with your feelings.

We may have typically witnessed that when a woman goes through heartbreak she cannot even touch food. In fact, the thought of it makes her feel sick. Alternatively, you see in movies or adverts girls munching their way through chocolates washed down by wine. How about when you first meet a potential partner and out of sheer excitement, you literally can't eat and the pounds drop off (for the wrong reasons)? This is an obvious clichéd example of how food is connected to our emotions and state of mind, but the above scenarios are those I'm sure at some stage we can all relate to. Your personal relationship with food and your emotions may be more subtle, of course, yet it is important to be aware that it has a powerful impact. Some people do use it as a crutch.

One of the most important exercises to practise when you are struggling with a food attachment or obsession is to simply express your feelings. If you can, find a good empathetic friend who will listen to how you are feeling. By simply talking about your feelings you are letting go of emotion. It is even better if you can lend a sympathetic ear to someone going through the same experience. In that way, this takes you out of your own self-absorbed head-space of constantly obsessing about food and also helps another person. While you're helping someone else, you're literally healing yourself.

If you are not ready to share and open up, it is really important to have a space where you can let go of how you are feeling. Perhaps you could speak to a professional therapist or mentor. You can even write it down to let it all out. I use breathing methods similar to the yoga ones previously demonstrated in this book and breathe it out of my system.

Remember, suppression leads to depression. I used to find on days I isolated myself, I would eat more as I wanted to push all the feelings back down. Most people think that pushing down feelings will make them go away and they hope they'll never have to address them again. You're not saving your health like this. In fact, you're doing exactly what you don't want and making yourself more susceptible to disease. Pushing emotions down will make these emotions manifest in the physical body and subconscious. Next time they come up, they will be even bigger and have more detrimental effects on your health.

Think about food allergies, for instance. We are fine eating a certain type of food, then suddenly we develop an allergy for no apparent reason. Well, it isn't for no reason, it is usually all connected to our emotions. Our bodies find it hard to break certain foods down because our digestion is lacking in creating the correct enzymes. Why is this? Our stomach area is connected to our feelings. Think about the last time you were really excited and how we describe the feelings of having 'butterflies' in your stomach. What do butterflies feel like?

How about when we are very stressed and nervous and develop IBS (irritable bowel syndrome)? From my experience, all allergies and food disorders are the 'red herrings'. Underneath them all is a big sea of emotion that needs addressing. Treating your allergy only will not make it go away for good. Feeding yourself temporarily treats the symptom in the short-term and doesn't even start to touch on the root cause. Yet again it's a form of masking. Just as you would throw a tablecloth over a table to hide the scratches, when you take it off again the scratches would not have magically vanished.

Once you start to unravel the layers to get to the core, you will experience a rollercoaster of emotions. While you're at this stage, sit with whatever you're feeling. Sometimes I used to feel strong as I wasn't using food as my crutch any more, however, if I found it easy to give up one compulsive behaviour, it was usually because I moved onto another source for my fix. Don't be fooled by this. That is why it is important to face the emotions and accept them even if it feels really uncomfortable. Eventually, through this process of surrender, you will come out of it stronger and liberated.

When you eat a meal, eat consciously. Today's rushed, fast-pace 'grab a sandwich' lifestyle, does not serve our health and digestion very well. When you eat with awareness your body will tell you when it is full. Listen to your body and respect what it tells you. In fact, your body is always talking to you, but are you listening? It takes at least 20 minutes for your body to register that you have eaten, therefore slow down. If you're overstuffed and still want to shove more food in, ask yourself, what is going on for me emotionally? Sit still for a second and tune into how you're feeling. Remember to put a full stop after each meal when you are three-quarters full.

If you're out in a restaurant and have finished your meal quicker than everyone else, ask the waiter to take your plate away or if there is some food left on the plate (even though I'm not a believer in wasting food), saturate your plate with salt and pepper to avoid picking at it until everyone else has finished eating.

Having a relationship with food and a poor self-image can really set you up for being out of control. The more you feel you are controlling your food and figure, the more it is controlling you. Learn to let go, accept and love yourself.

Remember to apply your positive affirmations when you are shifting away old energetic ways of thinking and use them as your power tools to stay on track for mind discipline.

# Delicious smoothie recipes

Smoothies are a quick and simple way of supplementing your diet while getting all the benefits of the nutrients being absorbed into your body instantly. They can be used by athletes, super-mums and dieters as a meal replacement and are a fantastic way to build up the immune system.

When making smoothies use, ideally, organic ingredients. You must drink them straight away to get the full nutritious benefits. Carrying around the smoothie all day in a container is going to let all the goodness of the vitamin, mineral and enzyme content diminish further. Therefore to take full advantage of the supplementation a smoothie gives, drink it as fresh as possible.

Remember to have a mixture of carbohydrate and protein for balancing the blood sugar. All too often, smoothies can be full of only fruit sugars, which can play havoc with your body's sugar levels. If you mix your smoothie with a form of protein, this will help stabilise the blood sugar levels and not give you a sugar rush followed by a dip afterwards.

These smoothie recipes are literally sufficient as a whole meal as it includes your carbohydrates, proteins and fats.

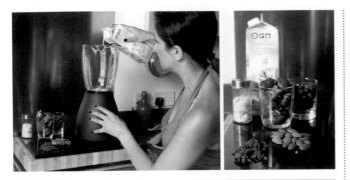

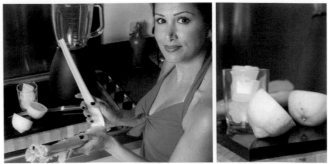

## Very berry smoothie

▸ Half cup (8 tbsp) blueberries

▸ Half cup (8 tbsp) strawberries

▸ One scoop of hemp protein

▸ Small handful of goji berries

▸ One small handful of almonds

▸ Half cup (4 fl oz) soya milk and crushed ice

Place all the ingredients into a blender, whizz until smooth and drink immediately. This is a great energy booster for after a work-out or as a nutritious snack.

## Detoxifying smoothie

▸ One whole large peeled cucumber

▸ 3 stalks of celery

▸ Juice of half a small lemon

▸ ¼ teaspoon of freshly grated ginger

▸ Small cup of ice

Juice the cucumber and celery in a juicer. Squeeze out the juice of the lemon and put all three ingredients into a blender with the ginger and crushed ice. Drink this first thing in the morning to give your liver a cleanse.

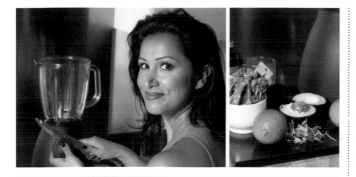

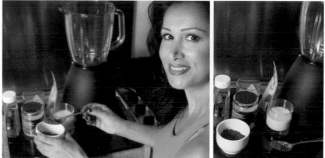

## Green smoothie

▶ Half a large avocado

▶ One cup (I small head) of broccoli

▶ 2 tbsp of freshly squeezed lime juice

▶ 2 tbsp of EFAs
(essential fatty acids, omega 3, 6 and 9 oils)

▶ 5 leaves of fresh mint

▶ Half a cup of crushed ice

This delicious smoothie is rich in nutrients and as you're juicing the broccoli, the beta carotene from it is fat-soluble, therefore your body will absorb it more efficiently, increasing the health benefits. Remember, these types of fats are 'good fats'. Your body and hormones in the brain will use them for energy as opposed to storing them like hard fats such as cheese, butter, etc.

After you have juiced the broccoli and squeezed the juice of the lime, add all of the ingredients into a blender with the crushed ice.

## Raw chocolate smoothie

▶ 2 heaped tbsp of cocoa powder

▶ Half a cup (4 fl oz) soya milk

▶ 1 tbsp agave syrup

▶ One handful goji berries

▶ One tsp coconut oil

Mix all these ingredients into a blender for a real quick pick-me-up. This smoothie is fantastic if you crave chocolate. If you cut down on the soya milk to less than half, and use cocoa butter by melting it first, you can put this in the freezer and have your own supply of raw chocolate.

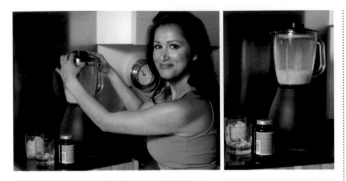

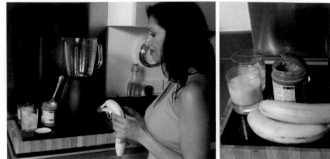

## Alkalising smoothie

▸ ¾ tsp of wheatgrass

▸ Half a cup (small bunch) watercress

▸ 4 small carrots

▸ Half a cup (4 fl oz) almond milk

▸ Half a cup of crushed ice

Make sure you juice the carrots first and then add all the ingredients into a blender. The wheatgrass is full of chlorophyll, which is created from direct sunlight and nature's most health-promoting nutrient. This is the best living superfood supplement one can find. Wheatgrass has 90 out of 102 of all the vitamins, minerals, enzymes and amino acids needed to get a balanced diet. Personally, I can't live without this. If I need a quick surge of energy I make a quick shot mixed with water. This smoothie will also help bring the body to an alkaline state. Alkalinity gets rid of acids, therefore eliminating fats which the body holds on to.

## High energy smoothie

▸ 1 tbsp of peanut butter

▸ 1 banana

▸ Half a cup (4 fl oz) soya milk

▸ Half a cup of crushed ice

Put all the ingredients into a blender and have this smoothie if your feeling tired or need a pick-me-up snack before exercising for supplying you with optimum energy.

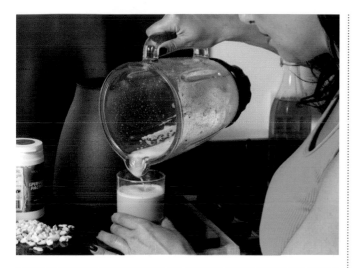

## Power protein smoothie

▸ 2 tsp spirulina powder

▸ 3 tbsp natural bio yogurt

▸ One handful unsalted cashew nuts

▸ Half a cup of crushed ice

Place all the ingredients into a blender, blend and drink immediately after a work-out. This is a great recipe for getting a good boost of protein and aiding in healthy digestion. Spirulina is a blue/green algae which grows in water. It is classified as a superfood, which has all the essential amino acids and vitamin and mineral content we require. It is natural, digestible and a good probiotic.

Enjoy your smoothies!

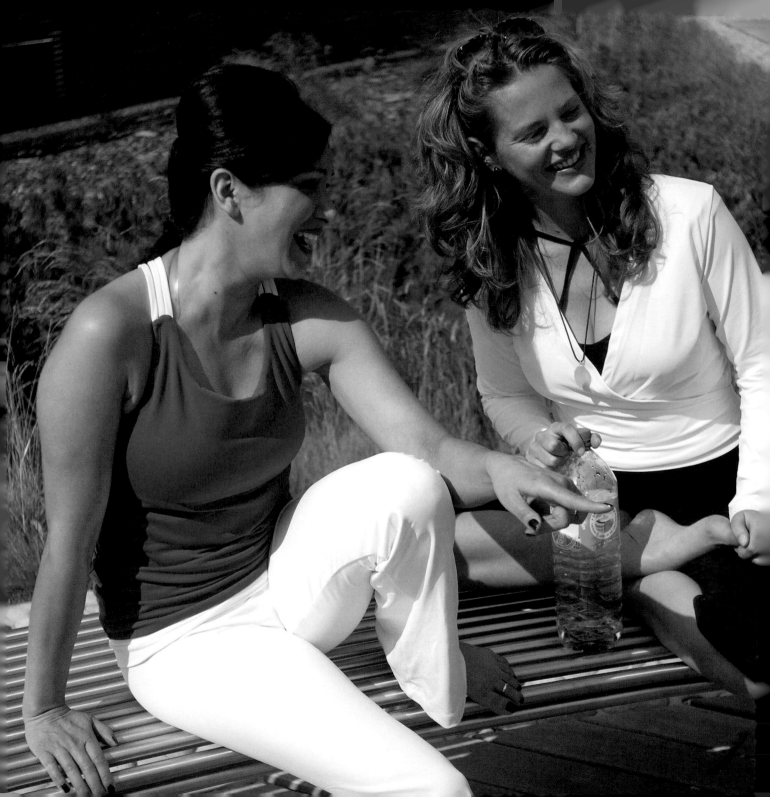

# Conclusions

**Life is a magical journey if you let it be.**

To learn to have success on every level in your life is all part of the journey because success is not a destination.

Never be put off by the harsh judgement of others. My personal message to all those judges out there who are fuelled by ego is: your days are numbered. When you stop judging yourself, you will stop judging others. When you start accepting yourself, you will accept others with their faults and all. If you expect nothing and accept everything in life, you will never be disappointed.

Remember, always follow your dreams because your dreams don't have deadlines!

Never assume someone else is smarter than you!

Finally, I would like to acknowledge myself and thank myself for always being my own rock and my own best friend! All I ever had was my sense of self-belief and faith. The universe did the rest of the work for me. I am humbled with gratitude and feel truly blessed.

*May all beings everywhere be happy and filled with peace.*

Loka Samasta Sukhino Bhavantu

# Testimonials

'I would like to comment on your class – I came across this by chance, and after two children and not having the time to get to a gym this was a godsend. I have been doing your class, three to four times a week for nearly a month and already can see and feel a great difference in my body. I have even increased my weights size from 1.58–2kg (3.5–4lb) to tone more. The abs section is my favourite! I can now actually see my abs prominently and everyone comments on how great my stomach looks, which has increased my confidence no end! Your inspirational talk throughout the class constantly reminds me throughout the work-out, even when I'm tired, to come back to the original goal and think of the results. Thank you Ladan, I owe my new-found body shape and confidence to you.'

*Emma Marlow from Eastwood, Nottingham, customer care specialist*

'Your work-out is simply brilliant and is dramatically changing my body. I had an awful jellylike bit on my tummy from having a baby and just haven't been able to get rid of it. Slowly but surely it's starting to tighten up and it's so exciting! I used to have a lovely flat tummy and I've so missed it! So once again, thank you! PS, I cannot believe that you are 40! Thought more like 29 or 30... Wow!'

*Angelina*

'I find that Ladan's work-outs have given me great results in helping me to lose weight and tone my body. They have also inspired me to keep up my fitness routine because they are full of variety and vigour. Ladan's classes show you ways to help train not only your body and muscles but your mindset too, and all while keeping it simple and fun to do.'

*Sharon Stroynowski, Data Manager*

'Thank you for being such an inspiration. I've never been a slim girl and really had a fight with my weight since childhood. I'm now in a position where I have lots of time free to be able to go outdoors and enjoy exercising. I'm reading your website and following you on Fitness TV and I really hope once I've changed my mindset towards food and exercise I will be able to lose the weight. At 23 I stand at 5ft 7.5in and weigh 13 stone (82.5kg)!! Ideally, I should be 10 stone (63.5kg)! I hope in four to five months time I can message you again and tell you I've lost three stone (19kg)!'

*SJ*

'I've been following your work-outs on Fitness TV. You've been amazing and I can already feel the difference in my fitness levels. Great website too. Thanks so much. You're a true inspiration.'

*Helen Dunne*

'Ladan has been my instructor for a number of years. I've been very fortunate to have known her, she's very professional and caring with a great sense of humour. Ladan's classes are very effective, you know you are always in for a treat, never the same and far from boring. After every single class, I feel my arms look more toned or my waist is smaller. Ladan has the ability to make you feel good about yourself.'

*Hashemi*

'Ladan has really changed my life. I went through a bad time with depression and stress for a number of reasons, but discovered her show on Fitness TV and her yoga/breathing techniques. They have really helped me improve and change the way I look at things for the better. She has a lovely warming personality that really comes across and helps to soothe. I can't thank her enough for the way she has helped me and influenced my life for the better. She has been a true inspiration.'

*Brett*

'Never before have I experienced such a motivational fitness professional as Ladan. I've always struggled to stay interested in strengthening and toning exercises. But, Ladan's driving force – a mix of inspiring, interesting and varied exercises, as well as her deep knowledge and sense of fun – means I never want to miss her class.'

*Charlotte*

'Two words to describe Ladan Soltani – "simply brilliant"!'

*John Hodges*

'I can't believe this young lady is 40? Are you sure? Wow, I would love to know your secret! I am going to be addicted to exercise and healthy living if I can look like you!'

*Sima Derrani*

'I love participating in Ladan's classes. She is not only a professional role model but I think her positive attitude and inspiring comments during her work-outs motivate me to keep going. This is a very powerful teacher who has taught me mind discipline and really cares about her class participants. Through attending her regular yoga sessions, I have seen a huge change within my body and mind. Thanks so much Ladan and keep up the wonderful work.'

*James Dougal*

# Testimonials (continued)

'I would like to take a few minutes to tell you my story. It's a simple one… but it's a good one!

I am a 50-year-old grandmother. I spent an entire youth, young adult life and fully grown adult life eating whatever I wanted with little or no consequence – even after the birth of my children. At most I would gain about five pounds and lose seven to make up for it!

Then, about five years ago, I began to notice that I was gradually becoming less and less fortunate! Slowly I realised that I was running out of luck. And worse, that I had no idea how to approach a good eating and fitness routine since I had never needed such disciplines in the past.

So, like most women I pushed the chore of my fitness to the back of my mind and pretended that I would get a grip on my diet and do something about it... soon... eventually... after the holidays!

I half-heartedly looked into fitness DVDs, toyed with joining a gym (actually, I've had two memberships and shamefully only attended approximately three sessions in five years) and then I gave up all together since, by this time, I had convinced myself that menopause was looming and that all my efforts would be a waste of time anyway.

And that's when I found you! I was looking for an advertisement and inadvertently came across you on the fitness channel. What caught my eye was your specific exercises for specific problems (ie lower body or upper body work-outs or aerobics and fat-burning). I liked that you focused on problem areas without all the dancey-dancey nonsense. Incidentally, not everyone wants to boogy the fat away! Some of us just want to burn it off with middle-aged dignity!

Now, don't get me wrong, it was no great earthshaking, thunder-clapping revelation! I still watched two of your programmes before I got off my mid-life crisis and decided to take part.

But taking part was the best thing I've ever done. It's been two months now and three of your programmes a week and I'm fitter than I have ever been! Even my husband of 30 years has noticed that I'm doing something... and has commented on how good I look and how firm I am! And this is a man who sat on a couch for a month before he realised it was new!
I love how easy you make it. I love how private it is. I love that I can have your personal attention at any time, day or night (I recorded your programmes) and that you make the hell of exercising a little less hell-like. I will keep up the routine and face menopause with a much better frame of mind... and a much better frame.'

*Anne de Bondt*

'Ladan Soltani has been such a positive influence in my life. Her kind words of wisdom have helped me enormously. I have experienced some life-changing shifts and always look forward to sitting in a meditation session with her and calming my senses. I owe you and thank you.'

*Kate Anderson*

'Hi, I think you're a great teacher and very entertaining. I am loving the results. Thanks so much!'

*Jasmine Sheen*

'I have to say, I've just started following your work-outs recently and already see a dramatic difference to my body shape and fitness! Thanks Ladan!'

*Janice Morgan*

'Your work-outs on Sky TV are really amazing. I've been following them from the start and my body has changed shape nicely. Keep up the good work and thanks.'

*Hannah Price*

'Ladan Soltani is my mentor! Absolutely fantastic!'

*John Harrogate*

'I want to thank Ladan for my new body and mind.'

*Silvia Kenning*

'We have been going to Ladan's classes for about two years now and love working with her. Whether it is a high-energy fitness class or a more spiritual (but equally challenging) yoga session, Ladan is always an inspiring and uplifting teacher, and she is also great fun. We always look forward to her classes. She always makes her classes lively and varied, but she also makes us think about what we're doing and makes sure we get the most out of every hour we're working out. After Ladan's yoga classes especially we always feel stronger, more relaxed and even serene – which is not easy with the busy lives we lead.'

*Kim Patel and Jane Upperton*

# About the author

## Business

Ladan qualified in London in 1990 as an Aerobics Director/ Personal Trainer. She began her career as an Aerobics Teacher specialising in a variety of classes including: step, high/low impact aerobics, aqua, body sculpt, circuits, body pump, aeroskip, boxercise, stretch, street dance, FitKid, 50+ seniors, core stability, yoga and meditation.

In 1993 she was headhunted by Phillip Wain International, a chain of prestigious health clubs in Asia. The success of her teaching and studio management in Hong Kong led to her obtaining a position as fitness director on board various luxury cruise liners where she was travelling and teaching around the world.

Ladan has now established herself as a recognised and highly sought-after fitness professional in London, where she personally trains high-profile celebrity clients and also teaches classes on a freelance basis for most of the exclusive health clubs. Ladan's energetic and motivating classes have a great following due to her infectious energy and her outgoing personality. Her work-outs are in huge demand and this popularity has led to both fitness clothing sponsorship from USA Pro and her own fitness chat show on the radio.

Currently Ladan is presenting on Sky Television for Fitness TV, where last year the viewers voted her the best presenter and her work-outs are regularly featured as the most popular on their homepage.

She's also a freelance fitness expert, writing for magazines and online fitness sites such as boots.com, AOL.com and *Health* magazine. Ladan has also had her work-outs published for *Health & Fitness* magazine. She provides regular features and work-outs for them on the latest state of the art training.

Ladan is also a fitness model and has a 'legs, bums and tums' work-out DVD with Fitness TV.

Fabulous Fitness at 40 is also available as a DVD work-out. Ladan has produced a TV series of this book and DVD for bodyinbalance well-being Sky channel. This series will be broadcast on many global networks around the world.

Ladan's exciting journey of living a healthy lifestyle, has now led her to the field of weight-loss, NLP and life coaching, as well as becoming a holistic nutritional therapist.

Ladan says, 'I love and live this lifestyle, so what an amazing opportunity to teach and share my knowledge and experience by helping other health-conscious, like-minded people to transform their lives positively. A healthy mind and body is the best gift you can give yourself and that is a fantastic investment in your life!'

## Personal

Ladan's personal journey of self-transformation has been explored on many levels. Apart from the fact that she was a young professional dancer from the age of ten, she has always been physically fit and she has immensely developed herself.

She started her professional fitness, dance and drama career in 1990 at the age of 19. This was the time she felt her first shift: she had discovered exercise and how good and confident it made her feel. At the same time, in this period of her life Ladan was always battling with body and weight issues. Unfortunately, this got unbearable and forced her to work on herself through seeking professional help and personal development.

From the age of 24 she has gained a great deal of knowledge, wisdom and emotional intelligence. She developed a strong urge to want to learn and understand existential psychology and was also curious about subjects such as addiction and compulsive and destructive behaviour, doing a great deal of self-study.

Ladan says, 'I believe we have three ways of being. One is the image we portray to others, the second is how others perceive us and, more importantly, the third is who we really are. My passionate search for answers bigger than myself lead to asking the big question as to why I was here on the physical earth plane.'

Ladan found a massive shift started happening when she discovered meditation seven years ago. It was the height of transition of divorcing her old life and entering a new phase of being. Her first experience of meditation was very emotional, profound and auspicious, and taught her to live outside the box in which we have been conditioned in our society today. She explains, 'I still meditate religiously every day. If I'm time-poor, I still make it a priority and then I wonder, "will I make it to my next appointment on time?" However, for some bizarre reason, when I'm rushed that particular day and still committed to dedicate a time to sit still, there happens to be no traffic. This is when you live in the magic of life and know that time has no concept. In fact, it is merely a creation of our mind.'

> ## Remove time from the mind and time no longer exists.
>
> Eckhart Tolle

This new paradigm of my life, compared to my past where I had no choice but to learn everything the wrong way without boundaries, has secured a sense of discipline and grounding within myself. It has trained and taught me how to sit with my feelings and accept them so that I can let them go and be free. These periods of what I call 'growing pains' were very dark and uncomfortable for me. However, I had to learn to surrender and connect to a universal energy source which was much bigger than myself. I also learned that I am not in control of anything in my life and that this bigger divine energy is always there guiding me to all the wonderful opportunities and privileged spiritual gifts I have been given.

My biggest polar change happened after my life-changing experience in India in 2007. It may sound like a cliché that I came back newborn and saw the world in a completely new light, however, this really was my personal and incredible experience.

I went to the Himalayas for eight weeks and for four of those weeks I trained as a 'Sivananda' yoga teacher, living on an ashram (Indian religious retreat with a monastery type of lifestyle) and participating in regular spiritual practice. This really taught me to live in the present moment and pushed me to places way out of my comfort zone. These days living out of my comfort zone is when I feel most alive. In fact, I crave that opportunity as I know for sure I will grow and gain a great deal from the experience. Unfortunately at the time, I resisted it and blocked the rewards which would have been given to me had I been more open.

During my time in India, on the last day of my course to be precise, I remember vividly sitting at the top of the ashram overlooking the stunning mountains of the Himalayas while crying like a baby. It was at this time that I had an emotional cathartic purge and regurgitated a lot of old painful feelings which had manifested themselves and lived in my body for a very long time (perhaps even before this lifetime). Literally I played back traumas and times in my life when I had felt really hurt by people and identified with all the times I had hurt others. It all came up and was left out to dissipate and dissolve into wonderful nature, and my whole being felt cleansed and purified.

When I came back to the UK after India I was never the same person. I felt at one and aligned with the cosmic consciousness. I became aware that everything which happens in the macrocosm is in me, the microcosm. My pranayama (yogic breathing) and meditation practice became deeper and my mind had astronomically expanded.

## *We need meditation not medication.*

### Ladan Soltani

Initially, I couldn't understand how one-by-one everything I had dreamed of started falling into place. Then I had an epiphany and understood that by diminishing everything in conjunction with the ego and only working from the heart I had shifted my energy. In the past I used to feel drained by others trying to take my energy and sometimes after teaching, being as fit as I was, I would still feel so exhausted after a session that I had to go to sleep to recuperate. I realised that if you are helping someone selflessly without any expectation, then no one can take your energy; on the contrary you should feel energised. If you feel drained and tired in a job where you are helping others, then you still have an attachment to ego and want something in return. Doing it from a place of sincerity and authenticity is extremely satisfying and rewarding.

Eight months after my India trip, I decided to take another course, this time in Ashtanga yoga, on an ashram in San Francisco. As I was aware of what to expect, this time I did not resist it and remained open. Well guess what? It was after this course that I discovered my life purpose, and I knew I had found my vocation in life. I cannot tell you how liberating this was for me. Knowing why you're here and what you are supposed to do is illuminating and enlightening. I know I'm here to help people wake up physically, emotionally, mentally and spiritually, and to acknowledge that there is a lot more than the 'material world' in which we live.

This does not mean I disagree with the luxurious things in this material plane, however, my personal interpretation of having the finer things is simpler. What it means is that your true core essence as a human being should lie with how wholesome and real you are. Material things should not validate us. True strength comes from a person who can live with or without these 'goodies'. If you take them away, ultimately one should still find an organic happiness within, without the superficial objects which supposedly qualify our joy.

To further my knowledge and training even more, I took a course in NLP (Neuro-Linguistic Programming), hypnotherapy and time-line therapy. Nowadays, I help people as a weight-loss coach, mentor, nutritionist, personal trainer and TV presenter. I help and motivate my clients to achieve their fitness goals through all the practices I have shared with you in this book. In order to help others I have found that fusing all my qualifications and experiences together has created a powerful package.

I always live my life following and listening to my intuition. My intuition is my biggest guide and most reliable friend. It is so accurate that it can almost feel surreal. When I'm not sure about something I sit and ask for the answers. I see my angels when I need them; they reveal themselves to me in specks of glistening, shiny, bright light. I have the gift of seeing coloured auras around people and see many spectrums of light every day. Light is all around us, yet not everyone has trained their eyes to see, even though we are all capable. I have gained these abilities through silence, retiring into solitude with a regular meditation practice and staying in good shape.

We all have a magnetic field of energy around us called the aura. The aura shifts and changes in colour depending on our mood and what is going on in our life or what is coming in. It is subtle energy which vibrates on a different frequency to matter.

When you meditate you become very aware of other frequencies. A great metaphor to demonstrate this; do you remember record players? Well if the needle was really sensitive what would happen? First of all it would pick up every single sound on the record due to its sensitivity and highly sophisticated needle. Second, all the dust would gravitate towards it and finally, you would have to put a small coin on top of the needle to ground it. This is the same theory with meditation; it makes you so aware and sensitive that you can pick up information about people just by being in their company.

Personally, I can usually get a good insight into a person if you mention their name and show me a picture. People gravitate towards you when you are living in light. It teaches you to connect to yourself including others and your surroundings. I feel very calm in my mind and relaxed in my body after meditation. I find you gain clarity and see things much more clearly. When life is fast-paced and speedy you lose that clarity and miss the stillness and beauty. Fast pace is like turning up the volume on a stereo to maximum and all you hear is a distorted sound. Naturally I am an anxious person who can, if not present or conscious, get lost in the crazy, chaotic world. Through my pranayama and meditation practice, I have learned to slow down and acquire a great deal of wisdom.

> *When I'm praying or chanting, I'm talking to what I call the divine universal energy. Yet, when I'm sitting silently in my meditation practice, the divine universal energy is talking to me.*
>
> Ladan Soltani

I still feel like a novice and continue to have a hugely driven appetite and knowing for the occult, esoteric philosophy, spirituality, mystical theologies, law of attraction and metaphysics. I am forever searching and passionate about helping. I have realised through my search, that the more I know, the more I realise I don't know!

The wonderful part is that I have met and attracted like-minded people. I have fantastic friends who are compassionate and supportive and they have become a part of my soulful community. When you have positively influential friends in your life, appreciate them and treat them like rare jewels.

Embrace life as though it is a gift. Treat others the way you wish to be treated and be kind to yourself and others. The universal law of karma is always alive and will come back another day in another way regardless of how you're conducting yourself. When you're being good to others, you're being good to yourself.

I really hope you have enjoyed my book and found it motivating and inspiring. If it has even woken up one person, that is enough to start a change.

> *Be the change you wish to see in the world.*
>
> Mahatma Gandhi

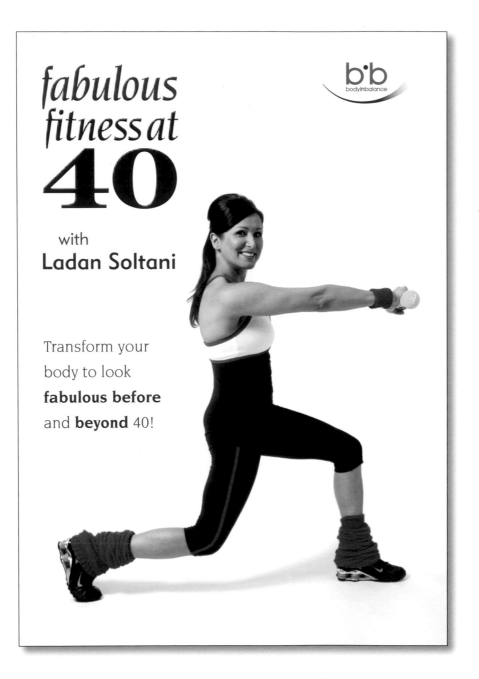

*fabulous fitness at* **40**

b·b
bodyinbalance

with
**Ladan Soltani**

Transform your
body to look
**fabulous before**
and **beyond** 40!

A DVD to accompany this book is available now for £14.99 from **www.ladansoltani.co.uk**